ROUTLEDGE LIBRARY EDITIONS:
SLEEP AND DREAMS

Volume 6

THE SLEEP INSTINCT

THE SLEEP INSTINCT

RAY MEDDIS

Routledge
Taylor & Francis Group
LONDON AND NEW YORK

First published in 1977 by Routledge & Kegan Paul

This edition first published in 2018
by Routledge
2 Park Square, Milton Park, Abingdon, Oxon OX14 4RN

and by Routledge
711 Third Avenue, New York, NY 10017

Routledge is an imprint of the Taylor & Francis Group, an informa business

British Library Cataloguing in Publication Data
A catalogue record for this book is available from the British Library

ISBN: 978-1-138-23090-3 (Set)
ISBN: 978-1-315-10370-9 (Set) (ebk)
ISBN: 978-1-138-23222-8 (Volume 6) (hbk)
ISBN: 978-1-315-31289-7 (Volume 6) (ebk)

Publisher's Note
The publisher has gone to great lengths to ensure the quality of this reprint but points out that some imperfections in the original copies may be apparent.

Disclaimer
The publisher has made every effort to trace copyright holders and would welcome correspondence from those they have been unable to trace.

Ray Meddis
University of Technology
Loughborough

The sleep instinct

Routledge & Kegan Paul
London, Henley and Boston

First published in 1977
by Routledge & Kegan Paul Ltd
39 Store Street,
London WC1E 7DD,
Broadway House,
Newtown Road,
Henley-on-Thames,
Oxon RG9 1EN and
9 Park Street,
Boston, Mass. 02108, USA
Set in Times Roman
by Weatherby Woolnough
and printed in Great Britain by
Lowe & Brydone Printers Ltd, Thetford, Norfolk

ISBN 0 7100 8545 1

Contents

Preface

Swimming against the scientific mainstream is, at the same time, thrilling and frustrating. This book describes and argues for a theory which not only runs counter to current medical thought but also challenges what appears to be good common sense. The theory is that sleep serves no important function in modern man and that, in principle at least, man is capable of living happily without it. The thrill of working with such a theory is that it amounts to a revolution in thinking about an important human process - not just a simple step forward. The frustration is that progress in convincing others is inevitably slow. However strong the arguments, scientists and laymen do not lightly dismiss the wisdom of centuries.

Nor do I take arms against such formidable opposition without some trepidation. When the theory first took shape in 1967, it was given only occasional public airings before audiences who might be critical but not hostile. Perhaps, some elementary mistake had been made. Perhaps, I had overlooked an obvious argument which others had not felt important enough to make explicit. As time went on, it became obvious that this was not the case and new evidence arrived every month to confirm my opinions.

Latterly, I have found that I am not alone. Bernie Webb, a respected elder statesman of the sleep-research world, has independently drawn conclusions which match my own. These are tentatively summarised at the end of his recent book, *Sleep, the Gentle Tyrant.* We do not agree on everything but we are united in one essential belief - that sleep has important non-recuperative functions in animals which may no longer apply to civilised man. For the first time, I begin to feel that the gap between myself and the establishment is not so wide.

In the chapters which follow, I have presented the arguments, as I see them, in favour of the new perspective. I hope that they will provoke a reappraisal of your own views rather than a stone-wall defence. A new theory of the function of dreaming sleep is also given. This is much more speculative and, once again, I find myself offering a formulation which is the direct opposite of established orthodoxy. Not only do I believe that dreams offer no survival advantages, but the suggestion also is made that dreaming sleep is positively dangerous and has had to be reduced to a just-tolerable minimum in man, other mammals and birds. Once again, I am tempted to apologise for being preposterous but again you will find that orthodox thinking has accepted a theory before there is enough evidence to justify anything more than an hypothesis.

I am indebted to the university system which makes available the time and facilities for the conception and nurture of such theories. The exercise has been enjoyable. I hope, in the last analysis, that it will have been worth while.

1 The joy of sleep

Like a great river flowing through a city, the sleep instinct flows gently but powerfully through our lives. While we can do nothing to stem its flow, we can and do come to terms with this natural force by sacrificing to it one whole third of our life. Indeed our sacrifice is often an enthusiastic one and sleep is rated by many as one of the greatest pleasures of life. They look forward to bedtime and savour the hours spent in bed until they reluctantly get up in the morning. Not everyone takes this view, of course. Many yield daily to the pressures of sleep without giving it a second thought until something goes wrong, like having difficulty in falling asleep. Like many pleasures, sleep can be easily taken for granted.

It may seem strange to talk about sleep as a source of pleasure rather than simply as a response to a felt need but if you doubt my proposition that people look to sleep as a source of pleasure as much as they look to good food, good company, wine, women and song, then try the following experiment. Ask yourself how you would respond to an (imaginary) new pill which would banish forever the need to sleep. I stress that this pill would cause you never again to feel drowsy, never again to nod off, but even so you would experience no ill-effects from the lack of sleep. Be quite clear, however, that once you have taken the pill you will never ever again fall asleep nor experience the desire to do so.

At first, you will probably be intrigued by the prospect of an extra eight hours of wakefulness which could easily be put to good use. You may enthuse about no more bed-making, no more wasting time getting ready for bed and later getting dressed again and no more early morning blues while shaking off tiredness before getting up. Perhaps you may think of taking another job or using those extra hours to write a novel or study for more qualifications.

But then you will wonder whether you really want to be active for twenty-four hours a day. It's nice to put your feet up in the evening, even to lie down in a soft warm bed. Bed is a convenient place for love-making and how sweet it often is to fall gently and happily asleep afterwards. After a long day with difficulties on all sides it is pleasant to switch off and forget, to relax and take it easy, to discard all responsibilities till tomorrow.

In the end I shall find few takers of this non-sleep pill. Admittedly sleep is a nuisance but with careful management it does not interfere too much with a full and happy life. On the other hand sleep is too much of a joy to be separated from for ever. The same is true of sex which can also be a terrible time waster and source of limitless anguish. Yet, if we offered a single pill which would remove sexual desire for ever how many takers would we find? Sex like sleep is a potential source of pleasure which few wish to see taken away whatever difficulties its presence may otherwise cause.

Whereas the pleasures of sexual gratification are readily identified and analysed the matter is nowhere nearly as simple in the case of sleep. How can we say that we enjoy sleep when we are in fact unconscious at the time, apparently unaware of anything? Certainly people do not smile often during sleep and in the morning they rarely recall much of their experience. At first sight it looks to be a proper paradox.

It only remains a paradox if we insist on thinking of sleep as the same thing as being asleep. Usually when people say that they enjoy their sleep they are talking about more than simple unconsciousness. Sleep refers to the whole ritual of going to bed, slipping between the inviting covers, relaxing with closed eyes, drifting off to sleep and even the joy of waking at six in the morning to the discovery that you have another whole hour before needing to get up. The pleasures of sleep are not those of unconsciousness but the appreciation of being free to go to bed, free to drift off to sleep and, if we wake during the night, free to fall asleep again.

The parallel between sleep and sexual gratification extends beyond the potential for pleasure to the possibility of pain when either urge is frustrated. Here lie the miseries of insomnia and prolonged sleep deprivation. When we go to bed drowsy and hopeful, it is painful, and for some agonising, not to be able to fall asleep. During the night it can be intensely irritating if we wake up and find that we cannot get back to sleep. If this pattern continues night after night, the frustration and irritation can build up to depression, general misery or hyper-irritability even though (as in sexual frustration) there is no direct damage to health.

Another painful feature of sleep is the nasty business of getting up in the morning. Some lucky people do not experience thick-headed, irritable reluctance but they are in the minority. The man who discovers a marketable potion which causes us to wake up cheerfully will also have discovered a fortune. It has always seemed strange to me that the nausea we feel on waking after eight hours sleep is so similar to the nausea of prolonged sleep deprivation. Perhaps they are similar because in both cases we are highly motivated to go back to sleep.

Sleep as a motive

The desire to sleep is a motive which can be just as strong as the desire to eat or drink, even though psychologists rarely include it in their list of drives. A motive can be weak at some times and strong at other times; sometimes we are hungry, sometimes we are not. At any given time there is a competition among motives and it is the strongest one which gains control of our behaviour. In the evening when our desire to sleep is low and our desire to watch television is high, we watch television. Later our desire to sleep becomes more intense. At some point it becomes greater than our interest in the television and then we get up and go to bed.

Motives reflect the brain's ability to control our behaviour by changing our priorities. In the case of hunger it is fairly clear how this works. When our food reserves fall low the brain detects this and makes a number of internal adjustments so that food becomes more attractive. If our hunger is not competing with some other more pressing need then we engage in learned sequences of activities which will bring us into contact with food. After we have eaten a certain amount the brain will adjust our priorities so that the food becomes less attractive and we will be tempted to get up from the table and set about some other more attractive project.

We shall need to consider how the sleep motive works in

particular but first we should see how the satisfaction of a motive is linked with pleasure and pain. It is tempting to think that the pleasure associated with hunger comes with a full belly but this is too simple an analysis. Consider a hungry man driving through a fog to a restaurant where he knows that he can eat well. He experiences pleasure at a number of points, for example when he first sees the restaurant through the fog, when he gets into the dining-room and discovers that he is not too late for dinner, when the food arrives at the table, when he tastes the first delicious mouthful and finally when he experiences that warm glow of relaxed satisfaction at the end of the meal. Pleasure, it seems, is experienced at each of the signposts *en route* to his ultimate goal.

Alternatively pain may be experienced whenever he meets a signpost which indicates delay or frustration of his intentions, when he discovers that he is too late for dinner, when he notices that the waiters are serving other customers before him, when the food he tastes is obviously undercooked and when at the end of the meal he finds that he has not had enough. Pleasure and pain are the two guides which keep us on the narrow pathway to consummation. Pleasure encourages us when we are progressing well. Pain or displeasure discourages us when we stray from the quickest route to final satisfaction.

This analysis helps us understand why the pleasure we associate with sleep need not be experienced while we are actually unconscious. Instead it occurs at the various landmarks on the road to sleep. For some reason the brain decides in the late evening that being unconscious is an important goal. In order to achieve that goal it adjusts our priorities and creates a sleep motive which will make sleep-related achievements more pleasurable and other achievements less so. At this time it becomes pleasant for us to lie down, sweet to close our eyes and delicious to drift off. After that it does not matter. The goal of the sleep motive has been achieved, unless, of course, we wake up during the night and then it becomes pleasant to fall asleep again.

The sleep control mechanism

One of the brain's many jobs is to assign priorities, to decide which problems will be tackled first. Sometimes it is fairly obvious how these decisions are made. The sight of a pretty girl has the effect of intensifying the courting urge, often at the expense of our desire to drive carefully. An empty belly gives food-seeking priority over studying. What, then, causes the brain to assign a high priority to falling asleep?

It is tempting to assume that the desire to sleep arises from the fatigue associated with prolonged waking activity. In other words the brain knows when it has had a hard day and needs a good rest. This is certainly a most popular belief but for two good reasons we should be suspicious of so simple an answer. First, no one has succeeded in showing satisfactorily that physical or mental effort is related to a need for sleep,[1] and second, observation of people who fly across time zones on long journeys has shown that the brain decides when to be sleepy on the basis of body-time, i.e. the time it *thinks* it is.

Because we feel tired at bed-time it is most natural to feel that we sleep because we are tired. The point seems so obvious that few have ever sought to question it. Nevertheless we must ask, 'tired of what?'. It is true that people feel tired at the end of a hard day of manual work but it is also true that office workers feel equally tired when bed-time comes. Even invalids, confined to beds or wheelchairs, become tired as the evening wears on. Moreover, the manual worker will still feel tired even after a relaxing evening in front of the television or reading a book which we might reasonably expect to have a refreshing effect. There is no proven connection between physical exertion and the need for sleep. People want to sleep, however little exercise they have had.

Perhaps the desire for sleep is related to mental fatigue. Once again we shall find that there is little proven association. If anything, sleep comes more slowly to people who have had an intellectually challenging day, possibly because their minds are still full of thoughts when they eventually retire. Ironically a quick way of sending someone to sleep is to put him into a boring situation where the intellectual stimulation is minimal.

There is no good reason to believe that our sleep motive is aroused so that the brain can have a rest. Many people have suggested that during sleep the brain clears away waste products which have accumulated during wakefulness, or manufactures new chemicals which will be needed during the next day. So far this is still little more than biochemical fantasy supported not by evidence but by the preconceptions of scientists who have been educated to believe that sleep is necessary for some kind of physiological repair process to take place. So far, everything we have learnt about the brain indicates that it could continue indefinitely, like the heart, without any pause for refuelling. Studies of nerve cell activity during sleep show that individual cells can be equally active during both sleep and waking.

Observation of long-distance travellers suggest that the desire for sleep is triggered more powerfully by the time of day the brain thinks it is, rather than by the length of time since they last got out of bed. For example, an American from New York visiting England on a business trip may have to leave his hotel bed at 7 a.m. every morning in order to keep to his appointments schedule. If he normally retires at 12 midnight at home in the USA, he may attempt to do the same in England but, during the first week at least, he will discover that he is not really sleepy until 5 a.m., i.e. midnight New York time. Because he has to rise soon after, he will be living on very short sleep rations indeed. Neverthless he will typically find during these first few days that when midnight comes he is wide awake and not yet ready for bed.

These considerations suggest that on a normal day the brain promotes the sleep motive to a high priority at a certain time, irrespective of what has happened during that day. At this time, activities preparatory to sleep are made to seem especially pleasant. If for some reason we do not yield to the lure of bed, then the priority increases gradually over the succeeding hours. It is this gradual increase after bed-time which creates the illusion that the critical factor, which triggers the sleep motive, is the number of hours of preceding wakefulness. Under normal circumstances however, the sleep-control mechanism is guided by the time of day (as judged by the brain) when choosing to create the predisposition to sleep.

Sleep as an instinct

Man is not the only animal in creation to spend many hours each day in a state of semi-conscious immobility. Far from it; sleep appears to be the rule rather than the exception in the animal kingdom. It is, in fact, so common that many authors have been tempted to think of sleeping as instinctive behaviour. Roughly speaking, an instinct is an innate biological force which predisposes the organism to act in a certain way. Instinctive behaviour is automatic and involuntary. Moreover the behaviour pattern is very similar in all members of the same species. This certainly appears to be true for man. In any large city, between the hours of 11 p.m. and 1 a.m., there are millions of people all rubbing their eyes and yawning, all saying how tired they feel, all making their way to bed, making themselves comfortable, closing their eyes and lying still. The action patterns are automatic, stereotyped and largely involuntary.

Instinct theorists usually divide instinctive actions into two phases. The first phase is preparatory and technically named 'appetitive'. In the case of the sex instinct, the *appetitive phase* is the courtship period. The second phase involves the actions which constitute the goal of the instinct; this is called the *consummatory act.* Copulation and ejaculation are consummatory acts. As for the sleep instinct, the appetitive or preparatory phase includes all actions which contribute to getting us comfortably settled into bed, whereas the consummatory act is the business of falling asleep.

There is still considerable controversy attached to the idea of instincts. Many believe that the concept is not at all helpful in understanding the control of behaviour and we shall do well to avoid this particularly tangled argument. Let us note, however, that authors often use the term instinct to emphasise that the major components of the behaviour pattern are largely genetically pre-programmed. This in turn suggests that the behaviour is vital to the survival of the species. Individuals are therefore born with the capacity and the predispostion to act in this particular way when the circumstances are appropriate. Some learning is often required but very little is left to chance. As a result, almost all adult male animals raised in natural surroundings will copulate effectively given the right circumstances. Similarly, they will all make their way to the appropriate sleeping site and fall asleep at the right time of day.

If sleep is an instinct, we might speculate that it plays a vital role in the survival of many species. It is certainly largely unlearned although it does slowly come to be associated with a large number of learned habits. Whereas sexual behaviour is typically stimulated by the sight or smell of a receptive partner, sleep is not obviously affected by external influences. Instead the sleep instinct is triggered by an internal clock which registers the time of day. Once triggered there follows a fairly regular sequence of actions which, with a little luck, is soon followed by the consummation of sleep.

The idea that sleep is an instinct, which is stirred everyday at a particular time, is a radical departure from the traditional view that sleep is a passive response to the accumulated fatigue of the day. It reflects a growing tendency among scientists to reject the idea that sleep is a passive state. Increasingly they see sleep as a state which is actively switched on, and later switched off, by some central control mechanism, like the urge to hibernate which many animals experience when the days grow short and cold. Long nights and inclement weather do not directly make these animals sleepy. Instead they trigger some central mechanism which sets in motion all of the action sequences which prepare for the long period of inactivity. Only when this appetitive phase of the hibernation instinct is complete, can the consummatory act, of falling into the long sleep, take place.

Drowsiness

The view that sleep is actively controlled by the central nervous system has one very surprising but important implication. This is that our feelings of sleepiness which we experience in the late evening are artificially created at that time by the brain and that they need bear no obvious relationship to the activities of the preceding day. It is as if the brain has decided that it is time to go to bed.

It is a pity that the recent intensive sleep-research effort has almost totally ignored the magical phenomenon of drowsiness. It appears quite spontaneously and grows insidiously from an imperceptible beginning to become a powerful force in a matter of hours. Like most feelings it defies verbal analysis but you may care to reflect upon its nature when drowsiness comes over you tonight. The physical components of this feeling are particularly difficult to specify but a mild itching of the eyes which causes rubbing is obviously common. At the same time a conscious effort is required to keep them from closing. Many people feel a kind of muscular itch which makes them want to stretch. This is accompanied by muscular reluctance which increases our awareness of effort when we begin to do things. Rubbing the eyes and stretching the limbs brings only temporary relief and the symptoms return quickly. The conviction grows slowly but certainly that the only solution is to close the eyes, lie down and rest.

The most striking aspect of drowsiness is the way it changes your attitude to what you are doing. Whether you are reading a book, watching television, enjoying a conversation, filling in a crossword or whatever, your interest gradually slackens. You are unlikely to fall asleep on the job but your ability to maintain concentration and your inclination to continue, gradually weaken. At the same time the idea of lying down in a warm bed becomes more and more attractive. How quickly the change takes place depends upon the interest of the task in hand. Drowsiness quickly takes over if you are reading a boring book but it can be held at bay for hours if you are having a good time at a party. Sooner or later, however, we yield to the attractions of the supine posture and the freedom to close our eyes. Sooner or later we end up in bed.

Drowsiness is the chief agent of the sleep-control system. It is used not only to get us to bed but also to help us fall asleep. If we wake up during the night, drowsiness is still there to help us gently back into unconsciousness. It helps us fall asleep by causing the mind to wander aimlessly, to drift about, in such a way that we do not notice our translation from the world of the waking into the underworld of the sleeping. Normally the brain abhors the possibility of falling unconscious and resists it vigorously. During advanced drowsiness, however, our thoughts are meandering elsewhere and this prevents us from being aware of falling asleep. Indeed, if we were aware of it we would automatically struggle against it. This is why rituals prescribed to counteract insomnia are usually designed to take your mind off the topic altogether.

Sustained concentration requires interest. We cannot concentrate on a book which we find boring. However hard we try, our mind cannot help wandering and it is often some time before we realise that our attention has slipped. Drowsiness works by lowering our interest in most things. This produces the characteristic difficulty we have in studying late at night and the lapses of attention observed in sleep-deprivation experiments. Our poor concentration interferes with effective performance and encourages us to give up and go to bed through the mechanism of frustration. It also lubricates the slippery pathway down into sleep by distracting our attention at the crucial moment of transition into unconsciousness.

The system is not so crude as to cause us to fall asleep suddenly at a set time. That would be too dangerous. We would run the risk of being caught short and rendered helpless in an exposed position if we were unable to get home in time. Instead drowsiness merely applies pressure to get us to go home and to go to bed. Only when we are settled will we fall asleep.

This leads to a complication, however. On the one hand the brain wants to succeed in getting us into bed, but on the other hand it must allow a certain amount of freedom to resist drowsiness if the situation so requires. What then is to prevent us from resisting drowsiness indefinitely if we so desire? This problem has been solved by using a compromise. Drowsiness is initially easy to resist but gradually it becomes more and more powerful, over a number of hours, to the point where further resistance is unpleasant.

This compromise is successful up to a point. On a normal evening if we are bored, we yield early by going straight to bed. If we are enjoying ourselves or doing something which we want to finish, we can delay sleep onset for a number of hours before drowsiness takes control. In a dangerous and therefore high priority situation we can fight off sleep for a number of nights. For example, in war-time it is quite common for combatants to go a number of nights without sleep. However, here the system breaks down because the deleterious effects of drowsiness upon efficient performance are such that they can be a serious liability. This is the direct result of the need to compromise between flexibility and firmness by the sleep-control mechanism.

This explanation of why we become more and more tired is a little different from the standard view which likens the sleep-deprived man to a runner who keeps on running or a hungry man who is continually denied food. According to the sleep instinct view, drowsiness increases according to a plan or stratagem whose aim is to get you to bed. It does not necessarily increase because our need for sleep is any greater. One of the advantages of the sleep instinct view is that it can explain why we feel more awake at 10 a.m. than 3 a.m. on those occasions when we stay awake all night. The early hours of the morning are the worst and you feel more and more alert as the morning progresses even though the number of hours of sleep deprivation are increasing.

The reason for this is that drowsiness is controlled largely by our internal clock system. When the time for waking up arrives, drowsiness is switched down to a minimum even if we have had very little sleep. Many people find that they have great difficulty in sleeping during the morning after a night awake. Of course there is a certain residual tiredness which becomes very obvious during the next day if we find ourselves in a boring situation. This residual tiredness results from the compromise discussed above. Its purpose is to prevent you from staying awake for a second night. It is usually not too troublesome during the day but on the second night the drowsiness can be overwhelming.

The purpose of sleep

To summarise, it is proposed that we all carry in our heads a sleep control mechanism whose action is timed by internal clocks which trigger off feelings of drowsiness and fatigue at certain times of day. This drowsiness increases slowly in intensity until it is strong enough to cause us to go to bed where it also helps us to fall asleep. If we wake during the period set aside for sleep, continued drowsiness causes us to fall asleep again. After the time set for sleeping has elapsed, drowsiness is switched off and we cannot fall asleep again even if we want to. If we yield to the pressures of drowsiness by going to bed and falling asleep, we shall experience pleasure. If we resist for any reason we shall experience discomfort.

It is natural to explain our feelings in terms of the experiences which have gone before. Therefore, it is typical to ascribe our sleepiness at midnight to the fatigue of our preceding labours. This tendency to refer our sensations to external causes may well be the main source of the traditional view that we need to sleep in order to recover from the exertions of the previous day. On closer inspection it is really quite difficult to make a strong case linking drowsiness with mental or physical fatigue. In general we find that the more relaxing and stress-free the evening the sooner our feelings of drowsiness occur and the more intense they are.

These considerations make it safer to conclude merely that there exists a powerful central-nervous-system mechanism which induces feelings of drowsiness and triggers sleep-preparatory behaviour at a particular time of day. Because it appears to be instinctive, we might presume that this mechanism is serving some purpose which is vital to survival. *This purpose, however, is as yet unspecified.*[1]

Of course it is tempting to say that we need to sleep to get rid of the tiredness we feel late at night. Strictly speaking that is true because if we don't sleep, then our feelings of tiredness will certainly increase. Such an explanation misses the obvious question of why the drowsiness was put there in the first place. Why does the brain make us feel drowsy? The answer to this question is equally simple. We are made to feel drowsy so that we will feel the desire to go to bed. The ultimate question now becomes, 'Why should the brain contain a mechanism which makes us go to bed for eight hours every night?'

This book sets out to answer that very question. Hopefully, it will be clear by now that there are some problems with the old idea that we sleep simply in order to rest. If it is not yet clear, then the following chapters will present some more evidence which aims to show that the traditional repair theories may be quite wrong, so wrong in fact that the time may have come to choose a whole new set of explanations.

2 The origins of sleep

> Although active during daylight hours there were occasional periods when a fish was buried under the sand or was inactive. Once darkness supervened, however, all fish became inactive, burying themselves completely or partially under the sand or laying against one another on the sandy tank bottom. During this state of inactivity they could be lightly touched without evoking an alerting response. On many occasions a fish could even be lifted by hand to the water surface before he became fully alert and swam off (Tauber, Weitzman and Korey on the reef fish, slippery dick).[1]

The discovery that fish sleep comes as something of a surprise to most people. Even sleep theorists have largely ignored the fact that the sleep which they are studying in humans is really quite common among remote animals. Moruzzi,[2] one of the most distinguished physiologists of our time, commits himself thus: 'Several lines of data suggest that sleep recovery is mainly required by higher nervous structures concerned with perception learning and maintenance of consciousness.' But the fish does not have any higher nervous structures in the sense which Moruzzi means. Moreover, it engages in precious little learning during its life time and I doubt whether the problem of 'maintenance of consciousness' is particularly troublesome to the slippery dick!

It is possible, of course, that sleep in the fish is different from sleep in man and we shall need to consider the point carefully. But we must always proceed with great caution when it is suggested that man is somehow different from animals. Darwin with his theory of evolution, taught us an important scientific lesson when he emphasised the similarities between man and his animal cousins. It makes much better sense to assume that sleep evolved to serve a simple but important purpose in animals and that it still serves the very same purpose in man. At least we must make this assumption until we are given a very good reason for thinking otherwise.

It is always flattering to think that sleep is serving some special purpose in us. It has been suggested that sleep helps to reprogramme our sophisticated computer-like brains. Alternatively, some reflect that it exists to permit some kind of emotional release to help sort out our tangled emotional lives[3]. Well, that is all very well but what about the simple-minded slippery dick? What purpose does sleep serve for him? What evidence is there, beyond wishful thinking, that sleep serves a different purpose in man? I would need a lot of evidence before I could accept that sleep was needed by fish for reprogramming purposes or for any kind of instinctual release.

Keeping out of trouble

Sleep is necessarily a spare-time activity. It has to be so because it can only be indulged in when all of the essential activities of life have been completed. Such activities include finding food and water, looking after young, grooming, mating and other social activities necessary for survival. It is clear from the fact that many animals sleep for long periods, that these essential activities do not occupy the full twenty-four hours of the day. Most animals can get done what needs to be done in considerably less time. The rest of the time is therefore spare. This raises the very important question of what animals should do in their free time.

Now the chief goal in life of all species is simply to survive to the next generation and the best advice available to animals with time on their hands is to 'keep out of trouble'. Keeping out of trouble usually involves keeping out of sight and keeping still. And this is precisely what the sleep instinct usually achieves. Most animals are driven by their sleep instinct to get well out of harm's way first, then, and only then, to lie down and after that to keep very, very still. Fortunately it requires no voluntary effort to keep still. While asleep we are not aware of what is going on around us. As a result, we are not tempted to respond to, or to investigate, anything which happens. In any case sleep is subjectively so pleasant that it would have to be very important to tempt any animal away from its comfortable sleep site. At the very least then, sleep serves the purpose of keeping animals out of harm's way for much of the time when they have nothing better to do anyway.

It is worth noting just how successful this hiding aspect of sleep really is, even among civilised people. Consider how often it is that you see people sleeping. You know that all of your friends do it but they are careful not to let you see them at it. It could be argued that we are very vulnerable, during sleep, to attacks of all kind but in practice that is simply not so because our sleep instinct takes care to make sure that we are hidden away from all harm before we ever fall asleep. If you think about it, the only people who normally see you sleeping are people who you would trust with your life anyway. If you had any reason to fear for your life, you would experience great difficulty in sleeping.

Let us call this 'keeping out of trouble' view the *immobilisation* theory of the function of sleep. It is a simple theory - perhaps too simple for many people - but it is very useful in explaining how sleep evolved and came to be an important feature in the life of most existing animal species. Animals who wander around or sit about conspicuously during their spare time will surely be caught and gobbled up sooner or later. Whereas, those animals who have a special instinct for hiding away at these times will be more likely to survive. It is not surprising therefore that the species which exist today - that is, those species which have successfully survived millions of years of evolutionary cut and thrust - nearly all sleep for long periods each day. It is not surprising because it is the habit of keeping out of trouble which has helped them survive for so long.

Sleep in animals

This argument hinges, of course, upon whether we can agree that species other than man really are sleeping. If we use the sleep of man as a model then we will have little difficulty in agreeing that sleep is a very common phenomenon among mammals (e.g. cats, dogs, mice, monkeys, squirrels) and birds. Most mammals spend long periods lying down with their eyes closed. Similarly many birds adopt the common roosting posture, where they stand with their eyes closed and their head tucked under their wing. As additional evidence we can point to changes in the electrical activity of their brains which are broadly similar to the changes observed during man's sleep.[4]

The argument only really begins to become interesting when we discuss sleep in reptiles. The reptilian brain is very different from the mammal or bird brain. Either for this or some other reason we typically find that the electrical brain-wave patterns in reptiles are different. As a result, the electrical activity of the reptilian brain cannot be used as proof that reptiles do sleep. It is true that resting (sleeping?) reptiles do show slightly different brain-wave patterns from waking reptiles, which supports my argument in part, but the changes which occur from the waking state to the sleeping state are not the same as in mammals or birds.

Anyone who reads Tauber's delightful description of sleep of the chameleon cannot, however, help but be convinced that lizards do indeed sleep.[5]

> In the hours before sunset, the animal typically settles on a branch, curls up his tail in watch spring fashion and remains still, though constant independent eye movements persist. During this presleep state the lizard will not attack insects and will even ignore those which alight on its body .... Shortly after sunset the circular eyelids close, the eyeballs are retracted and the animal appears to be asleep. Unless disturbed, the animal will generally remain in this position throughout the night.

That is about as close a description of sleep as one could hope for. It shows many features of the sleep instinct as we know it. It begins with a journey to a safe place, on a branch, where a typical resting posture is adopted. His stillness and disinterest in even readily available food show the chameleon to be drowsy. Finally, he closes his eyes, demonstrating a desire not to know what is going on about him and lies still for a long period of time from sunset to sunrise.

All the sleep symptoms are there and, as a bonus, they occur at a particular time of day. Like us they sleep at night when small lizards are particularly vulnerable. The temperature drops when the sun goes down and they are unable to prevent their own body temperature falling. When this happens their behaviour becomes sluggish and they are readily caught and eaten. If they wish to avoid this fate then they must get out of harm's way *before* the temperature falls, that is before sunset.

Larger reptiles such as the crocodile spend enormously long periods in a state of complete immobility which must not be confused with sleep. Indeed it would be foolish to take 'eyes closed' as a sign that it is safe to approach. Crocodiles use immobility partly to conserve energy and partly to give them the advantage of surprise if any hapless prey comes too near. Nevertheless crocodiles do sleep some of the time, so deeply in fact that it is safe to approach and even pick them up briefly. At these times, it can take a croc a long while to come alert. The sleep state can often be diagnosed by the position of the four legs (see Figure 2.1) If the animal is lying on its belly with all legs pointing backwards and none out to the side, then it is highly likely to be asleep - but proceed with care!

Frogs, toads, newts and salamanders have also been studied and shown to have long periods of sleep-like immobility. These animals belong to the class of amphibia. Amphibian species of various kinds existed on the earth for millions of years even before reptiles evolved. Like reptiles the amphibia so far studied show long periods of unresponsive immobility at particular times of day often in particular sleep sites. As long ago as 1914 the naturalist Leffler studied sleep in amphibia. According to Hediger,[6] a European naturalist, Leffler was

> convinced that there is a true sleep state among amphibia, in particular the Axolotl and that this state can be recognised by a specific sleep posture. When asleep they are suspended at an angle in the water with their forelimbs slightly spread. The tip of their tail is supported by the ground or some aquatic plant. By 9 p.m. about 30% of his experimental animals were asleep, by 10 p.m. about 75% and by 11 p.m. about 90%. Younger animals sleep more deeply than older ones. The sleep state is not only recognised by the animal's characteristic posture but also by physiological indications. They react

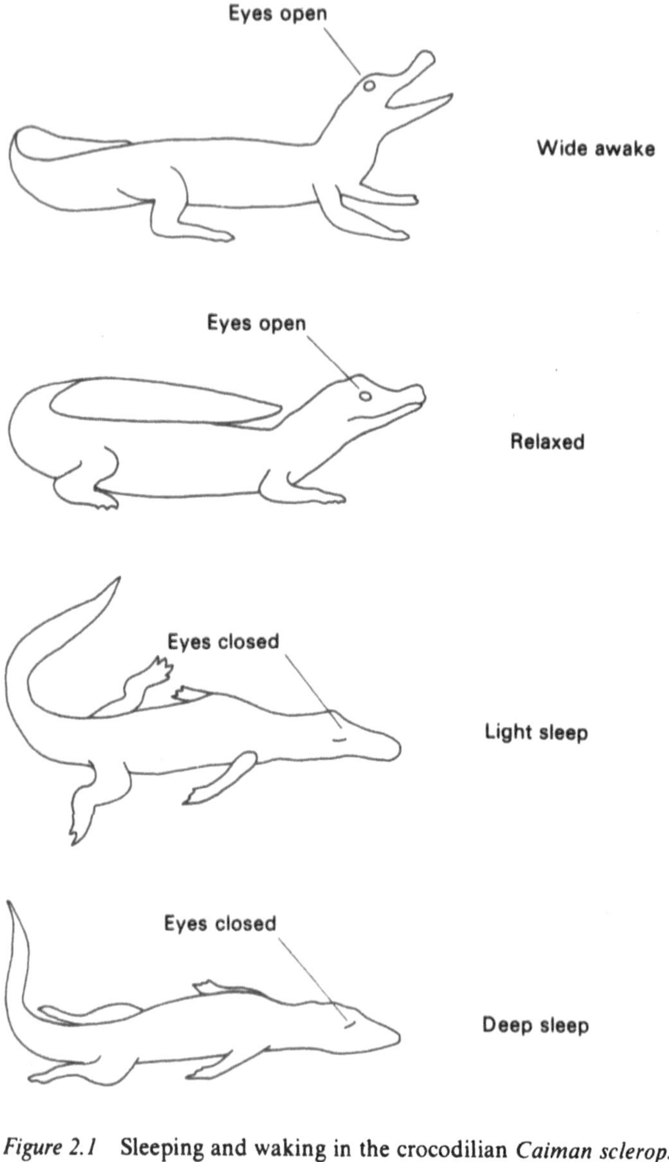

Figure 2.1 Sleeping and waking in the crocodilian *Caiman sclerops* (after photographs by W. F. Flannigan Jr, R. H. Wilcox and A. Rechtschaffen in Electroencephalography and Clinical Neurophysiology, 1973, vol. 34, pp. 521-38)

less or more slowly than when awake to light stimuli, to knocking on the aquarium and to direct touching. Above all we have almost certain evidence for the depth of their sleep in the frequency of their gill strokes. During sleep this falls to one per minute whilst normally it is an average seven per minute in otherwise similar circumstances.

We have already talked about sleep in the fish, slippery dick, and he is not alone in his night-time sleeping habits. Some species of parrot fish even wrap themselves in a slimy envelope during their night-time sleep. Tauber[7] also reports that 'gross observations made at the Bermuda Aquarium at night permitted one of us to observe the complete inactivity of numerous species of fishes as they were draped over or propped against rocks, or lying in the sand.' Peyrethon,[8] a French researcher, has reported on sleep in tench which sleep at the bottom of the tank all day. At these times the fish are slow to respond to disturbances.

Mammals and birds evolved from reptiles. Reptiles evolved from amphibia. Amphibia evolved from fish. Since mammals, birds, reptiles, amphibia and fish all show the phenomenon of sleep, we can be sure that it was invented, or rather it evolved, a very long time ago. Did it begin with fish or was sleep already present when fish evolved? Few people have directly studied sleep lower down the chain of evolution and we are largely dependent upon casual observations scattered here and there in zoological texts.

Molluscs, for example, have not proved favourite subjects for study among sleep researchers. One pioneer, Strumwasser,[9] has recently given us an account of sleep in the sea hare (*Aplysia californica*). These animals have no backbone and therefore constitute very distant cousins indeed to ourselves. Nevertheless, it retires every evening at dusk to a particular corner of the tank where it curls up into a specific sleep posture. It stays in this position until dawn, or just before, when it moves away to check its feeding dishes. It is then intermittently active for the rest of the day. Regrettably, no information is given about the responsiveness of the sea hare during these sleeping periods.

Insects, surprisingly, present very little problem when it comes to establishing the existence of sleep among them. Nearly all insects which have been studied show at least one inactivity period per day. During this sleep period they remain well hidden and out of trouble. Andersen,[10] a Danish entomologist, has studied responsiveness in the Mediterranean flour moth during sleep. Normally the lightest tickle will cause it to fly off but during sleep the contact has to be considerably more forceful. Wasps and bees sleep at night, presumably because they rely to a considerable extent on vision for their navigation. They sleep together in hives, holes in the ground or on a special sleep-tree or bush.

Perhaps it is going too far to suggest that the day-time torpor of the cockroach is the same as our night-time somnolence. Well, perhaps it is, but the general point is made that a basic pattern of sleep-like behaviour is present in at least insects, molluscs, fish, amphibians, reptiles, birds and mammals (including man). This pattern consists of a long period of inactivity and low responsiveness which occurs in a safe place at usually the same times each day. In fact sleep is a very common phenomenon among living things which possess the power of locomotion.

It is certainly true that this pattern shows variations in detail from species to species according to the particular needs of each. Sleep in mammals is undoubtedly more complex and varied than sleep in the mollusc even though the basic pattern is similar. Whilst it is possible that this increased complexity reflects some change in the function of sleep, I shall argue that in the absence of strong evidence to the contrary we must assume that the purpose remains the same but that an increasingly complex mechanism is required to achieve the same aims as the animal itself becomes more complex.

How much sleep?

Before we proceed much further, the idea that sleep is a spare-time activity will need a little clarification. For many animals there are times of day when it could be argued that there is little option but to be inactive. For example, many species of reptiles would be at a considerable disadvantage if they attempted to be active at night becuase cold-blooded animals operate very imperfectly when the environmental temperature falls. Similarly, most birds and bees share a dependence on daylight for their ability to navigate when flying. As a result, inactivity in a safe place is the best policy when the sun goes down, whether or not they are still hungry. In one sense, this is still 'spare' time because it cannot be put to any useful purpose.

The sleep instinct, because it is an instinct, operates involuntarily. The time for going to sleep and the time for waking up are programmed into each animal. The length of time asleep varies from one species to another but is very much the same for individual members of the same species. These schedules have been worked out carefully over the eons of evolutionary time to fit the particular life style of each. They might make life difficult for some individual animal but, for the species as a whole, they are delicately tuned for best effect.

Table 2.1 gives some indication of the variation of sleeping times among mammals whose sleep has been studied in detail. The estimates vary enormously from no sleep at all to twenty hours a day. It is certainly difficult to explain this variation in terms of differences in their metabolic or intellectual needs. Why, for example, does the sloth need twenty hours sleep while the guinea pig needs only eight?

Hediger[11] is alert to this problem and has suggested that the amount of time spent sleeping depends upon the life style of an animal and the security of its sleeping quarters. He contrasts the sleep of the lion and bear with that of the antelope. Bears and lions are fearless creatures who can afford to perform in a leisurely fashion all natural functions such as drinking, copulating, giving birth and rearing their young who are born relatively helpless. Bears and lions sleep deep and long. By way of contrast the antelope is, of necessity, a timorous creature. It drinks quickly, copulates rapidly and produces young who are able to walk within thirty minutes of being born. The antelope sleeps briefly, if at all, in the wild.

However, cats and mice have very different life styles, hunter and hunted, but they sleep for approximately the same time each day. This comes about because of the high security of the mouse's sleeping quarters. (Have you ever tried finding a mouse when it is asleep?) Although the mouse, like the antelope, is generally considered to be a timorous creature, it can afford to sleep for longer because of the additional security which it acquires when asleep.

Table 2.1 Estimated number of hours sleeping time per day for various mammalian species[12]

Hours	Species
24	
23	
22	
21	
20	giant sloth
19	North American opossum, big (and little) brown bat, water opossum
18	giant armadillo
17	owl monkey, nine banded armadillo
16	Arctic ground squirrel
15	tree shrew
14	cat, golden hamster
13	mouse, rat, grey wolf, ground squirrel, tenrec, phalanger
12	Arctic fox, chinchilla, gorilla, raccoon
11	mountain beaver, slow loris
10	jaguar, vervet, star-nosed mole, European hedgehog, patas monkey, galago, desert hedgehog, mole-rat
9	rhesus monkey, chimpanzee, baboon, red fox
8	Man, rabbit, guinea pig, African giant pouched rat, East American mole, pig, echidna
7	
6	grey seal, grey hyrax, Brazilian tapir
5	tree hyrax, rock hyrax
4	
3	cow, goat, Asian (and African) elephant, donkey, sheep
2	roe deer, horse

Whereas the general life style of an animal and the security of its sleeping quarters are important influences on how long and how deep an animal may sleep, both are secondary to the issue of spare time. Sleep can only be valuable to creatures which have more time available than they strictly need to carry out the various duties necessary for their own survival and the survival of the species. Some kinds of animals do not have many demands on their time and they are free to sleep almost all day. Others need to be busy nearly all of the time and therefore cannot afford to sleep no matter how brave they are nor how well hidden their sleep site.

Food collection, for example, is often a time-consuming chore. Our own diet is very rich in nourishment and we may have difficulty in imagining the problems of the large herbivore whose food is of relatively poor quality. To help us, the London Zoo Guide specifies that the diet of its cow elephants (smaller than bull elephants) includes 100 lb of hay, 2 lb oats, 2 lb maize, 4 lb locust beans, 4 lb biscuits, 10 lb carrots, 10 lb potatoes, 3 or 4 cabbages, some apples and oranges, a loaf of bread, 1 oz salt and sometimes some fresh leaves, bamboo shoots, dried fruit and cod liver oil. The guide goes on to say 'In order to obtain the same amount of nourishment a wild elephant would have to consume a much greater weight of food and it is not surprising that wild elephants spend most of their time feeding.'

In circuses and zoos where high quality food is readily available, the elephant does have a fair amount of spare time and is reported to sleep for up to five hours. In the wild the situation is different and sleep is a luxury which cannot often be afforded. I have never heard of an observation of an elephant sleeping in the wild. It is noteworthy that, even in captivity, the elephant has the ability to go without sleep for long periods if it has any cause for anxiety.

The general principle which emerges from this survey of the admittedly sparse data on mammalian sleeping habits is that *the time spent sleeping by a given species of mammal depends mainly upon the amount of time available for sleep.* Across species at least, sleeping time appears to expand to fill up an animal's spare time. By spare time is meant time which is not needed for other essential activities or which, for other reasons, cannot be used for these activities. In this way time can be classified as spare if an animal has already completed all the jobs necessary for survival or if it is too dangerous to carry them out even though there are outstanding needs.

Controlling sleep time

Many species of birds migrate to more polar latitudes for the rearing of their young. This is not simply because their nesting sites offer a richer supply of food – although this is often the case. Polar latitudes offer an even more precious advantage in the form of extended daylight hours. Most birds require a large amount of food which is time consuming to collect. When rearing a growing family the problem is more acute and the time taken to collect the food must increase alarmingly. Since birds are very often unable to gather food at night in the darkness, one solution is to move house to a place where there is less darkness.

This illustrates the fact that night-time is free time for most birds because little useful activity can take place then. As a result these birds engage in sleep-like behaviour for most of the dark hours. In the summer the number of dark hours is reduced and the time spent sleeping is correspondingly reduced. Their sleep expands and contracts in keeping with the available spare time.

Similar phenomena can be observed in times of emergency or stress when most animals sleep less. When danger threatens, the urge to sleep is greatly diminished. We have already mentioned this in connection with elephants who will remain awake all night if a stranger is in the vicinity. Similarly we have all noticed the same effect on nights before examinations, job interviews or public performances. We are reacting to these events as if they were immediate threats to our safety. Danger restricts spare time because we need to defend ourselves and this job lasts until the danger has passed.

Day-to-day changes in our life situation are, however, much less important determinants than the inborn tendency to sleep for a specified number of hours. These values appear to be fixed according to species. For example, the opossum tends to sleep for over eighteen hours every day largely because it is an opossum, because it was born with a sleep instinct which keeps it asleep for over eighteen hours. Danger, hunger and cold will certainly reduce this value but the effect will simply be a deviation from an inborn tendency to sleep for a long time. On the other hand, the nervous guinea pig sleeps normally much less and in a threatening situation will sleep for even less, if indeed at all, but never will it sleep for as long as the opossum, whatever the circumstances.

It is as if we all have a 'sleep-stat' within us whose setting is genetically determined. The setting specifies how many hours we will normally spend sleeping. This setting can be altered within limits to suit circumstances but when things are running smoothly the sleep-stat resets itself to its natural value. This natural value is fairly similar for animals of the same species with only minor deviations. For example, we humans sleep an average of about seven and a half hours and it is rare to meet people who regularly sleep for less than five and a half hours or more than nine and a half hours. Under exceptionally boring and stress-free conditions we can sleep much more and when the need arises we can go without sleep altogether for a night at least. However, when conditions are normal we drift back to an average in the middle range. These findings suggest that the setting of the sleep-stat is fixed. In the course of evolution each species has determined, through experimenting, the ideal amount of sleeping time. This value is then passed on through the generations as an inherited tendency to sleep for so many hours. In this way each animal knows automatically how long it ought to spend waking and how long sleeping, without having to rediscover the ideal value by trial and error.

The advantage of being asleep

We have already seen how it is that the life style of an animal necessarily limits the amount of time which it can spend sleeping. Within these limits, however, there is a strong tendency for evolution to set the sleep-stat as high as possible. This suggests that, during spare time, sleep has a number of advantages over waking in terms of survival. Recuperation is only one possible advantage of sleep and is alone insufficient to help us understand the enormous variation in sleeping-times among animals. It seems unlikely for example that the sloth needs twice as much rest as the chimpanzee. In addition we must consider additional advantages which make sleep such very good value that each species takes as much as it can afford.

One of the most striking benefits arises from the fact that most animals are well hidden and completely still during sleep. This means that the chances of being preyed upon by natural enemies are greatly reduced. Take the sparrow for example. For him the time of greatest danger occurs during the day while hopping about looking for food. He has a minimum of cover in which to operate and his fast darting movements make him easy to spot. At night however the opposite is the case. He is carefully concealed in his hideaway, making no movement nor sound, confident that he will survive at least until the next day.

The sparrow is dependent upon daylight because he navigates by vision. In many ways this is unfortunate because it makes life easier for his natural enemies. Some animals, however, navigate largely by smell or hearing, like the rat and the bat. This means that they can be active at night which makes life more difficult for predators. During the day, when they would make easy meat, they are fast asleep where no-one can find them. Certainly, in their case, the less time spent awake the better, if they are to live to a ripe old age.

It is frequently suggested that sleep is a most vulnerable state. A time when we are unconscious, when danger can creep up on us unawares. Perhaps it would be so if we slept just anywhere, but we don't. People and animals are most particular about where they sleep. The sleep instinct influences behaviour by causing an animal to seek out the safest possible sites where dangers from any quarter are reduced to a minimum. Many birds sleep on high ledges or on inaccessible branches. The rat and the rabbit retire down their holes. The fox retires to its lair. Gregarious animals herd together. The hippopotamus retires to the water. Only animals which have nothing to fear, like the gorilla or the big cats, sleep casually in exposed places. For the rest sleep is a time of concealment and hiding, of security not vulnerability. It will be suggested below that hiding away is probably the most important benefit of the sleep instinct.

An automatic sleep/wake scheduling mechanism is clearly valuable for those animals who need only a few hours of activity each day to carry out all essential activities. If the mechanism is well devised, it can ensure that they are awake for the best few hours of the day, the times when food is most plentiful and predators least able to catch them. For some animals there are some times of day when it is absolutely imperative that they should not be abroad. We have already mentioned the fact that most birds are unable to fly at night - at least near the ground - because they need light to see where they are going. This makes it imperative that they retire to a safe place before, not after, sunset and that they are not tempted to fly away, whatever the provocation, until after first light. Small, cold-blooded reptiles have a similar problem because they have difficulty in keeping their body temperature high at night when the sun goes down. As they cool, they become sluggish and vulnerable to predation. Like birds, they have much to gain from a clock-timed sleep instinct which gets them to safety before the environmental temperature drops.

Life is a continual struggle to stay alive. On the one hand, this involves an effort to avoid being killed. On the other hand, it involves the regular exercise of collecting enough food to nourish and repair our body tissue as well as to supply energy for other survival exercises. As a result, food and water are most precious resources which must not be squandered in needless activity. Sleep, in a very obvious way, reduces the waste of energy by discouraging violent activity which would waste energy. It does this by making sure that the animal is unaware of the stimuli which would provoke action. A sleeping cat does not chase butterflies because it does not know that there is a butterfly to chase. Moreover, the sleep instinct causes the animal to choose a sleep site which is warm and well protected from the cold and damp. The sleep posture is also carefully chosen to avoid needless waste of heat. The cooler it is the more tightly the sleeper curls up.

The human newborn baby supplies a fine example of the benefits of sleep. By remaining asleep for more than sixteen hours each day he must keep his energy requirements to a minimum and thus reduce the strain on mother's ability to supply his needs. But more important than this is the survival value of being inactive for long periods. Mother's job of caring for herself and her many offspring is made easier by baby's sleeping habits. It can be fairly said that baby sleeps to prevent mother from becoming exhausted.

If you doubt this, discuss the matter with any mother of two or three pre-school children.

A sleep instinct therefore heaps a variety of benefits upon those species which possess one. The benefits depend, of course, upon the species. For some, the conservation of energy is most valuable, for others the protection from predation is paramount, whilst for others the cardinal benefit comes from the timing element which helps them anticipate dramatic changes in the environment such as the onset of darkenss and a drop in air temperature. For any given species, however, the benefits are not fully understood. Until recently, students of animal behaviour have almost completely ignored sleep and the role it plays in the life of the animals they observe. As a result, we are still restricted to loose generalisations concerning how we think sleep ought to help. Zoologists are at long last taking a greater interest in this problem and we might expect some useful analyses of the strategic value of sleep in the not too distant future.

Sleep enforcement

In the meantime, we need to note three of the most relevant features of the sleep instinct. First, it influences an animal to withdraw to the safety of a sleep site where it adopts an energy-conserving posture. Second, it uses some internal clock arrangement to ensure that this withdrawal will occur at the time when it is most valuable. Third, by altering the consciousness of the animal it produces a state of relative unawareness which helps to keep the animal in its sleep site until the appropriate time for venturing forth again.

It is often claimed that sleep is a state of unconsciousness but this is, in fact, a most unhelpful description. It is true that animals are relatively unresponsive during sleep but this need not imply that they are unaware of their environment; far from it. Many warm-blooded animals can respond very quickly indeed if the trigger-stimulus is important enough. During sleep they are simply more selective when deciding what to respond to and what to ignore. It is, of course, a common observation among human sleepers that they can sleep undisturbed through the noise of aircraft landing and taking off but wake up quickly to the sound of a baby crying in another room or the gentle click of a teenage daughter's key in the front door lock when she returns late from an evening out.

To examine this phenomenon we carried out an experiment with sleeping student volunteers which involved quietly playing their name once every seven seconds until they woke and pressed a button. The name was recorded on a short audio tape-loop which allowed us to play the name either backward or forward. Of course it was unrecognisable when played backward but it was equally loud and gave us the opportunity of comparing speed of waking up to meaningful and non-meaningful noises. When the name was played normally a response would take about twenty seconds on average. However when the name was played backward the average delay was more than one minute.

The students had been originally asked to press the button when they woke during the night for whatever reason. We must therefore conclude that waking up is slower for stimuli which are less meaningful. However, the brain must be making a decision as to whether or not the stimuli are meaningful *before* waking up. The sleeping brain is therefore aware of the stimuli and can discriminate among them with a view to deciding whether to respond or not. The delay in responding is not caused by a lack of awareness but by a reluctance to respond unless the stimulus is important enough. This indicates that the usual lack of response by sleepers is caused by a reduction in the sleeper's motivation.

It is reasonable to assume that this drop in motivation affects not only responses to external events but also the willingness of animals to perform actions on their own initiative. Thus a sleeping animal needs to become very hungry or its bladder needs to become very full before it will stir itself to leave the comfort and security of its sleep site. This explanation of the sluggisheness of the state we call sleep agrees very well with the analysis of the state of drowsiness in chapter 1. It was suggested there that drowsiness influences individuals to retire by reducing their motivation to continue with other tasks and as a result impairing their ability to sustain concentration.

We describe sleep in terms of unconsciousness because we fail to remember our experiences during the night. In retrospect, a sleep period is a blank period. Of course, this need not mean that we were completely unaware of our surroundings at that time. Instead it is more consistent to assume that we were aware but that few memories are laid down at this time. It is well known, for example, that adults experience dreams which add up to approximately a hundred minutes each night. We know that they are vividly experienced and yet it is common to wake in the morning with no recollection of them whatsoever. Clearly the absence of any recollection for the events of the night cannot be taken as evidence that we were unconscious and experiencing nothing all the while. It is true that responding is suppressed during sleep, but it is most unlikely that we are also unconscious.

Conclusions

Sleep is an ancient phenomenon exhibited by many different types of animal. It is characterised by behaviour patterns which involve withdrawal to a safe place where, as the result of a dramatic drop in motivation, the animal remains immobile and unresponsive for a sustained period of time. This behaviour pattern confers on the animal a number of survival advantages including protection from predators, isolation from the inclemencies of the environment and a reduction in energy requirements. Whether it is *also* a time when certain bodily repair processes take place is another matter which will require further consideration.

3 Very short sleepers

In the last chapter we discussed the theory that sleep helps animals to survive by keeping them out of trouble and by reducing wear and tear during their spare time. This idea is not unfamiliar to students of animal behavour but is usually regarded as very strange by people who have thought of sleep mainly as a human activity. For them the restoration theory of sleep is usually more attractive. After all, man does not need to keep out of trouble during the night since he has the ability to create light and warmth and no longer walks the prairies in fear of predators. Moreover, modern man usually has lots of spare time which he uses for having fun not for sleeping.

Perhaps the purpose of sleep in animals is different from its purpose in man. Perhaps, but we must not forget that man is an animal and his mastery of the environment is so far still very short-lived, a few thousand years at the most. For most of the time man has lived on this earth, he has been just as vulnerable as many other animals to the dangers of darkness and his instincts were fashioned with this problem very much in mind. Since the desire for sleep is fixed by his genetic inheritance, any changes which occur would require a series of genetic mutations which might take many thousands of years. Moreover, non-sleeping could only become a dominant feature of man's make-up if the environment became hostile to, and eventually destroyed, people who indulged in sleep.

As we well know, long periods of sleep in humans are quite compatible with a long and effective life. Therefore there is no reason why evolution should cause sleep to disappear. Moreover the time involved is too short to expect any significant changes to occur. As a result, it is quite reasonable to assume that our sleeping habits are largely unchanged from the days of our prehistoric ancestors. It follows from the immobilisation theory of sleep that our sleep instinct was originally tailored for men who had a rather different life style from the one we enjoy today. In other words sleep, as we know it, is an evolutionary hangover.

One of the important consequences of the immobilisation theory is that sleep may no longer be necessary in modern, civilised, opulent man. Although he feels the urge every night to go to bed and remain there till the late morning, it is possible that the time spent in slumber is completely wasted. According to the theory, the drowsiness which he feels is not a reflection of a bodily need for rest; rather it is a symptom of the action of the sleep mechanism whose purpose is to manoeuvre him to go to bed, to keep out of danger – danger which no longer exists.

Many people who have been convinced of the strategic value of sleep for animals, still insist that sleep could have recuperative value as well. This point of view is very attractive in many ways. Indeed we would expect sleep to acquire additional functions through the millennia. There must be many processes which are more effective if they occur while an animal is resting and as a consequence they will come to be confined to the sleeping period. The question which we must now ask is whether these processes could only occur during sleep. If we now removed sleep, would it prevent these processes from taking place? Has sleep slowly come to be physiologically essential?

To answer this question we simply need to take a healthy individual (human or non-human) who normally sleeps for a substantial proportion of the day, switch off his sleep instinct, by some means or other, then stand back and wait to see if he is disabled by this procedure to any significant extent. It sounds simple enough and indeed it may be possible in the not too distant future. Just at the moment we do not understand the circuitry of the brain well enough to make the necessary adjustments, although progress has been so rapid in recent years that we might confidently expect that the knowledge to enable us to go ahead will be available soon. It may require a brain operation or more hopefully a simple injection whose effects will be reversible. We shall have to wait and see.

Trying by an effort of will, to stay awake is not a sufficient procedure.[1] Sleep-deprivation experiments are simply attempts to fight the sleep instinct which responds always by fighting back with weapons too subtle for effective resistance. The vigilant volunteer becomes a battleground where we witness an unequal struggle between the desire to stay awake and the desire to sleep. What we really need is a procedure to switch off the desire to sleep so that he or she never even feels drowsy.

For the present we must confine ourselves to a search for individuals who may have had their sleep instinct switched off or disabled either in the course of evolution or as a result of an accident to the brain. Certainly, in our discussion of animal sleeping we noted a number of mammals whose sleep needs seemed to be very low. Large herbivores such as elephants and antelopes are rarely, if ever, observed sleeping in the wild. However, we do know that elephants and cattle do sleep in captivity when they are well fed and have little to fear. It is possible that these animals also sleep in the wild but that their vigilance is such that they hear us and wake before we see them. While it is clear that they usually sleep considerably less than we do, we must look a little further afield for better examples.

The Dall porpoise

Another intriguing report concerns the Dall porpoise, which, according to McCormick,[2] an American researcher, has never been observed to sleep. He studied ten captive Dall popoises and reported that sleeping behaviour was absent. He did not need to use recordings of the electrical activity of the brain because sleep in sea mammals is usually as easy to observe as sleep in man. The sea mammals which have already been investigated include dolphins, porpoises, whales and seals. All have been observed sleeping often for long periods - all, that is, with the exception of the Dall porpoise.

Sam Ridgeway and James McCormick have collaborated in experiments aimed at solving the problems of anaesthetising porpoises safely. As a result they have had ample opportunity to observe them sleeping naturally:

> A passive surface sleep has been described during which the porpoise hangs near the surface with the head and trunk almost parallel to the water surface and the tail dangling down somewhat. Both eyes are closed. In the absence of a water current the animal rests almost motionless. About twice each minute the tail will stroke slowly lifting the animal to the surface for a breath. Long periods of sleep (1 hour or so) are always of the surface sleep variety. . . . A second type of sleep referred to as 'cat napping' or 'bottom sleep' has also been described. In this type of sleep the animal rests near or on the bottom, coming up periodically to breathe. This napping may last as long as 4 minutes before the animal comes to the surface to breathe after which it may or may not resume the nap. A similar type of sleep behaviour has been noted in which the animal makes a few rapid swimming strokes and then coasts around the tank as its eyes droop.

It is clear that sleep in the porpoise is fairly obvious when it does occur. Moreover we may be confident that James McCormick is qualified to recognise it when he sees it. Nevertheless he has never caught any of his ten Dall porpoises napping. Ideally we would like to have his observation confirmed by round-the-clock studies of electrical brain activity. For the time being, however, we must consider the Dall porpoise as another serious candidate for our non-sleeper title.

Why the Dall porpoise should have different sleeping habits from other porpoises such as the well-known bottle-nose dolphin is very much a matter for speculation. It is certainly true that it is better adapted for deep diving in the sea and it is quite likely that it enjoys a very different life style from that of others. Perhaps it lives more dangerously. Perhaps its food supply is more time-consuming to collect. At present we simply do not know.

The swift and the albatross

There are other possibles which deserve the closer scrutiny of researchers. Among these we must include the familiar swift and the large sea-going birds such as the albatross. A number of birds have been studied in the laboratory including chickens, owls, pigeons, hawks and falcons. They all spend a considerable amount of time sleeping whether this is judged by their behaviour or by recordings of their brain activity. The swift and the albatross have not been so closely studied but we do have enough circumstantial evidence concerning their habits to make it appear extremely unlikely that they sleep under normal conditions.

The large sea-going birds are beautifully adapted to a life of almost continuous flying which involves few visits to land which rarely occur outside of the breeding season. Their wide wing-span takes advantage of the strong ocean winds to keep these birds aloft for the major part of their lives. The ocean supplies their food requirements and their airborne life style secures their protection from most predators. It is reasonable to suppose that these birds do not sleep on the wing since it would serve little purpose in terms either of resource conservation or of keeping out of trouble. If indeed they are able to sleep while flying, then this in itself is so surprising as to be worthy of special study, but it does seem most unlikely.

The swift provides an altogether more provocative illustration of a possible ability to keep out of trouble during the dark hours without recourse to sleep. There have been many reports which suggest that swifts congregate in the evening and then fly high into the air where they remain till next morining. Flocks have been observed flying at night at an altitude of approximately 5,000 ft by aeroplane pilots, and on at least one occasion a swift became lodged in the engine of an aeroplane so that positive identification was possible. This observation has been supported by radar studies.

It is reasonable to assume that the swift is safer when flying high in the sky than it would be roosting on the ground. According to the immobilisation theory there would be little additional benefit to be gained from sleeping while flying. Indeed it would appear to be a crazy thing to do. It is common, however, to read about the swift's amazing ability to 'sleep on the wing'. Such statements do not, of course, derive from any proof that they are asleep. Instead they derive from the belief that all animals must sleep because sleep is necessary for physiological repair processes. A perfectly circular argument! It would be nice to know one way or another whether the swift really does sleep while flying, but it does seem rather unlikely.

Nonsomnia in people

Even more interesting than sleeplessness in animals, is the possibility of finding a person who does not need to sleep. It is after all quite common to read newspaper articles about people who claim not to sleep. Is it possible that these characters are really telling the truth, or are they merely trying to catch a little publicity by exaggerating a tendency to sleep less than the average? If such people really do exist then they would constitute a strong piece of evidence in favour of the immobilisation theory of the function of sleep and they would propose severe problems for the old restoration theory.

Before we begin our search it is worth noting that we are looking only for people who are healthy and happy despite their non-sleeping. As such they constitute a quite different class of people from insomniacs who claim not to sleep a wink and suffer as a result. I prefer to use the term *nonsomniac* for people who sleep very little and who experience no desire to sleep any more. It is an important qualification that nonsomniacs are content with their short sleep and do not complain about it.

A good example of nonsomnia has been reported in various newspaper articles[3] which describe the case of Señora Palomino, a fifty-one-year-old Spanish lady whose home is in Caceres in the mountains south of Madrid. Her claim is not to have slept at all for thirty years. Her nonsomnia began at the same time as she dislocated her jaw (ironically by yawning). Although the jaw has since relocated itself her sleeplessness persists. She spends her nights sitting awake in an armchair. Not sleeping does not seem to be a problem for her:

> It doesn't stop her leading a very full life though. When she has finished her housework which begins at seven each morning, she runs a day nursery in her home for 27 children whose mothers go out to work. And nobody has ever had cause to complain that she does this responsible task in a sleepy-headed way.

The case is certainly most interesting. Señora Palomino appears to suit our requirements exactly. On the one hand she does not report sleeping while on the other hand she does not complain about the lack of sleep. As a bonus she lives an active and constructive life which suggests that her normal faculties remain unimpaired. If her case could be authenticated by sleep researchers, then we would have a perfect case of nonsomnia.

Alas this has not been done, and we must sympathise with sceptics who refuse to throw away their cherished beliefs merely on the grounds of newspaper articles. If we are to make any impact on the opinions of others we shall have to continue our search for an unassailable example. This really means that we need to lure a nonsomniac into the laboratory where proper checks and measurements can be made.

Two Australian short sleepers

A pioneer effort in this direction was carried out by Henry Jones,[4] an Australian doctor in Perth, Western Australia, in collaboration with visiting Scottish sleep expert Ian Oswald. They investigated the sleep of two healthy and active Australian men who claimed to sleep for only three hours per night. During one week of observations in the sleep laboratory they found that one volunteer, Mr Mck., slept for an average of 2 hours 47 minutes per night, while the other, Mr H., slept for an average of 2 hours 43 minutes.

For the purposes of the study, the two men were required to come to the laboratory in the small hours of the morning when they would be connected to an electroencephalogram (EEG) which measures the electrical activity of different parts of the brain. It is easy for a skilled technician to tell accurately when a person is asleep using the EEG record. While the measurements are being taken the volunteers lie comfortably in bed where they are free to sleep for as long as they wish. The procedure is not as disturbing as you might imagine and most people sleep as well in the laboratory as they would in a comfortable and quiet hotel room.[5]

Both were busy and successful professional men who found their nonsomnia of positive value in their private and public life. They volunteered no complaints of the kind often heard from insomniacs. Nor did they experience difficulty in falling asleep. In fact they had no sleep problems. The only difference between them and us is that they did not feel the need to sleep for longer than three hours.

Mr H. is described in the following terms:

> A 30-year-old draughtsman. His wife confirmed his story of sleeping only about 3 hrs. per night. He said that about 6 years previously he had decided to give up sleeping much because he was too busy.... He said that if he took holidays then he would sleep for more hours each night, but admitted that he had not actually had a holiday for some years. Occasionally he would take a nap of some minutes duration at the weekends. He is a civil servant but, in addition, keeps very busy by being the secretary of several Church and youth organisations. He does the secretarial and other organisational work for these during the night hours. He was a vigorous and over-meticulous man and not hypomanic.

Mr H. claims to have reduced his sleeping time 'because he was too busy'. At first sight, this may give rise to hope in many other business-men who find sleep a nuisance, but this may be a false hope. Mr H. also gives us some biographical information which suggests that his nonsomnia may be an inherited tendency. Apparently, his father had been a nonsomniac too, and often would not go to bed at all. Even so, father, like son, had maintained good health throughout.

The significance of this study, for our purposes, is that a dramatic reduction in sleep in certain individuals is compatible with health, happiness and effectiveness. Although these two men slept for only three hours each night, they cannot be said to be suffering from insomnia which is an unpleasant complaint. There was no conflict in them between the desire to sleep and an inability to get to sleep. They slept well enough but did not feel the need to sleep for very long. As we shall see, time and again, the most intriguing symptom of nonsomnia is the absence of any desire to sleep for as long as normal people.

Whilst these cases are undoubtedly very thought provoking, they could hardly be presented as evidence crucially in favour of the immobilisation theory and damningly against traditional restoration views. After all three hours is probably long enough for recovery to take place of whatever it is that is recovering. Nevertheless, I was encouraged enough by this evidence to set out myself in search of even more impressive cases.

A search for more nonsomniacs

The first step was to appeal through the media for nonsomniacs to come forward. This was a fairly easy matter because the press, radio and television keep up a steady trickle of items on sleep and especially insomnia. It was simply necessary to point out to reporters that not all non-sleepers were complaining and to encourage them to include in their report a request for such characters to write to me. In terms of the number of replies received, this campaign was highly successful. Unfortunately, the overwhelming bulk of the letters were from people who were really complaining about insomnia.

Many of the correspondents began by claiming that 'they never slept a wink' and then went on to supply enough information to assure me that they were getting at least six hours of sleep though probably of poor quality. Many told anguished tales of how they had switched from one sleeping pill to another with little or no relief of symptoms. It was clear that most of the letters had come from insomniacs rather than nonsomniacs and it was necessary to delete them from my list as courteously and sympathetically as possible.

Quite a number of letters, however, looked quite hopeful. These people were then invited to give me a detailed statement describing their sleep for two consecutive weeks. The questions asked included estimates of when they went to bed, when they fell asleep, when they woke up and when they got up. A depressing number of these statements, however, made it clear that my correspondents were getting considerably more sleep than they had originally said and they, too, were reluctantly crossed from my list.

A handful of replies did reflect sleep habits which were comparable to those studied by Jones and Oswald. For example, Mrs G. of Hertford sent me a detailed account of her sleeping for three weeks, during which time she appears to have averaged 3 hours 5 minutes per night. She is a retired district nurse and some extracts from her letter give a good impression of what nonsomniacs typically say about their sleep:

Dear Dr Meddis Aug. 15th 1972

Thank you for the form received which I will fill in and send to you when completed. This lack of sleep is a life long thing. I am sure I do not need a lot of sleep because I feel so well. . . . Also, I love night work because I do a lot of public speaking (as well as attending sick folk). I do all of my preparation during the night time. So long as I can keep my feet up I am resting. My background would make a good best seller. I am always watching people nearing the end of life and keeping awake is no problem at all.

Probably if I led a lazy life, I would doze off during the day but I can't be lazy. If I am not reading or sewing, I am gardening or sitting with an elderly lady near here whilst her husband goes shopping. The more I can help others, the better I like it, but I do prefer to do night work. . . .

Yours sincerely,
Mrs G.

Nevertheless, when all forms had been returned, there were very few people who were anywhere near the one hour maximum which I had set as the target for my study. One man, a Londoner, aged about seventy claimed to have had less than three-quarters of an hour sleep per night for the last thirty years. We invited him along to the laboratory for one trial night. He slept, according to our EEG recording, for 2 hours 22 minutes which, if kept up over a number of nights, would have been a record for the scientific literature but it was not nearly low enough for the purpose in hand. His sleep was very disturbed with five separate awakenings during this short sleep which added another two hours to the time separating initial sleep onset and terminal awakening. It was undoubtedly the case that these prolonged periods of wakefulness give him the impression that he had spent almost all of the time awake.

Our last hope was a fifty-two-year-old man from the north of England whose claim to have been an extreme nonsomniac since the age of sixteen evaporated in a single night in our laboratory. He slept for 5 hours 55 minutes! In the morning he persisted in his claim that he had been awake all night and regretted that we had not actually gone into the bedroom where we would have seen him awake. He had little faith in our EEG machine! Once again it seems likely that the illusion of not sleeping was caused by the nine occasions on which he woke up during the night. He spent 2 hours 57 minutes awake in addition to his sleeping-time and this must have given him the impression that he had been awake for the whole night.

Miss M.

At this stage the whole research project would have ground to a halt if it had not been for a casual reference by a friend to Miss M., a lady who, my friend claimed, slept 'for only an hour or two each night'. Rather half-heartedly we wrote to the lady and asked her to fill in the sleep report forms. By this time we had come to expect very little and we were very sceptical when we finally received her reply. According to her report (given in Table 3.1) she slept an average of only 49 minutes per night. The amount of time spent sleeping fluctuated markedly from night to night but never appeared to exceed 80 min. Had we really found a genuine nonsomniac? It seemed too good to be true.

At that time I was working in a team, ably assisted by Geoff Langford and Jo Pearson. Intrigued by her reply, we packed our tape recorder and set off from central London, where we worked, to a fashionable south-west London suburb where she lived. We were amiably received by Miss M., a seventy-year-old retired nurse, who cheerfully sat through a long recorded interview which allowed us to collect all the information we needed and to test her with all manner of questions designed to check whether she was not deluding herself on the matter. By the end of this session we were thoroughly convinced by the consistency of her story, but even then we had difficulty in bringing ourselves to believe in what is, after all, a most unusual phenomenon.

By her own account, Miss M. had been nonsomniac since childhood when she would spend the night reading books in bed while the household slept.

She was the product of a most difficult birth at which her mother died. Her father had already died during the pregnancy and she was brought up by relatives. She was born with a spinal deformity which prevented her from walking until she was ten years old and she still walks with a limp. Although she is a

Table 3.1 Sleep report volunteered by Miss M.

Day of week	Fall asleep - wake up	Time asleep
MONDAY	2.15 - 3.30 a.m.	(75 min.)
TUESDAY	2.30 - 3.45 a.m.	(75 min.)
WEDNESDAY	1.45 - 2.30 a.m.	(45 min.)
THURSDAY	2.50 - 3.30 a.m.	(40 min.)
FRIDAY	3.15 - 3.45 a.m.	(30 min.)
SATURDAY	2.45 - 3.30 a.m.	(45 min.)
SUNDAY	3.10 - 4.00 a.m.	(50 min.)
MONDAY	2.30 - 2.45 a.m.	(15 min.)
TUESDAY	3.15 - 4.20 a.m.	(65 min.)
WEDNESDAY	2.45 - 3.50 a.m.	(65 min.)
THURSDAY	3.30 - 4.10 a.m.	(40 min.)
FRIDAY	NO SLEEP	(- min.)
SATURDAY	2.50 - 4.10 a.m.	(80 min.)
SUNDAY	2.45 - 3.50 a.m.	(65 min.)
	Average	49.3 min. per night

Nights spent reading, writing, thinking

diminutive figure and has suffered much in her life, she is rebellious and tough by nature and never gives up without a struggle.

Like most other nonsomniacs, she is a busy lady who finds her ration of twenty-three hours of wakefulness still insufficient for her needs. Even though she is now retired she is still busy in the community, helping sick friends whenever requested. She is an active painter and has recently finished a biography of William Morris, the British writer and designer. Although she becomes tired physically, when she needs to sit down to rest her legs, she does not ever report feeling sleepy. During the night she sits on her bed (she never lies down) busying herself with reading, writing, crocheting or painting. At about 2 a.m. she falls asleep without any preceding drowsiness often while still holding a book in her hands. When she wakes about an hour later, she feels as wide awake as ever. It would be wrong to say that she woke refreshed because she did not complain of tiredness in the first place.

To test her claim we invited her along to the laboratory. She came willingly but on the first evening we hit our first snag. She announced that she did not sleep at all if she had interesting things to do, and by her reckoning a visit to a university sleep laboratory counted as very interesting. Moreover, for the first time for years, she had someone to talk to for the whole of the night. So we talked.

In the morning we broke into shifts so that some could sleep while at least one person stayed with her and entertained her during the next day. The second night was a repeat performance of the first night. Quite uninterested in sleep, she busied herself chatting and painting a miniature, and so on through the next day. By night three we were a little disorganised. Things had not gone according to plan. So far we were very impressed by her cheerful response to two nights of sleep deprivation, but we had very little by way of hard data to show others.

In the end we prevailed upon her to allow us to apply the EEG electrodes and to leave her sitting comfortably on the bed in the bedroom. She had promised us that she would co-operate by not resisting sleep although she claimed not to be especially tired. We left her at 1.00 a.m., leaving the light on so that she could continue reading and so that we could watch her on closed-circuit television. At approximately 1.30 a.m., the EEG record showed the first signs of sleep even though the light was still on and she was still sitting with the book in her hands. About one hour later she woke briefly, wiped her eyes, put the book down and soon after fell asleep again, remaining asleep for another 30 minutes. At this point she woke up suddenly and admitted to feeling confused and uncomfortable but otherwise she felt fine. She had no further interest in sleep and asked to be allowed to leave the bedroom so that she could join our company again.

On analysis she had slept for 99 minutes. Her sleep was not especially different from that of an average person. It contained dreaming and non-dreaming episodes and, as for other adults, the first dream was delayed for 60 minutes. The only substantial difference between her sleep and what we might have expected from any other seventy-year-old lady was that it was of shorter duration.

Since that first study we have conducted another survey of Miss M.'s sleep.[6] On this second occasion she came to the laboratory for a period of five days and nights. During this time she was watched round the clock by a team of mature girl students who volunteered to help us. During the day, Miss M. was free to travel and do what she wished as long as she was escorted at all times. At night she was prepared for an EEG recording whether or not she anticipated sleeping, and she was expected to spend at least two hours in the bedroom alone while we watched her on closed circuit television.

Throughout the week, Miss M. was alert and happy. She enjoyed the attention which was lavished upon her by the girls. As expected she did not sleep on Monday but she did sleep on all of the other days. Over the whole week she averaged 67 minutes per night which was near enough to her original claim of 49 minutes to remove any remaining doubts about the phenomenon.

In addition to our objective indicators of reduced sleep need, there are a number of other aspects of Miss M.'s story which fit the picture of the typical nonsomniac which has been emerging throughout the course of this research. First, she does not complain about the lack of sleep and would not appreciate being able to sleep more. Second, she does not report feelings of drowsiness either during the day or at night. Third, she demonstrates a robust personality with a positive approach to the problems of life. Fourth, she keeps herself busy and involves herself in the lives of others and the community generally. Fifth, she does not find anything strange in the fact that she sleeps for less than 20 per cent of the time normal people spend sleeping.

One further point is worth noting; Miss M. did not volunteer for the study, someone else put us in touch with her. Since meeting her I have made contact with other nonsomniacs and the mode of introduction has always been the same. Someone else has contacted me to tell me of the existence of a nonsomniac in their neck of the woods. On meeting the individual concerned I find that they do not find anything special or praiseworthy in their sleeping habits. It is simply the way they are. Nor are they keen to be paraded publicly as freaks – a reasonable sentiment which I hope the media will continue to respect.

I can illustrate the lack of concern for their sleeping habits by recalling a nonsomniac who rang a late-late radio phone-in on BBC Radio Newcastle. The show was compered by Ian Guardhouse and I joined him and his listeners on the appropriate theme of sleep. Our caller rang soon after 2.00 a.m. to discuss some war-time experiences, although we soon discovered that he was a two-hour nonsomniac. In the ensuing conversation we discovered that his mother was nonsomniac too. Encouraged we asked about the sleeping habits of his two sisters who lived nearby, only to discover that they had never discussed their respective sleeping habits! This reflects the general rule that, while non-somniacs are happy to tell you about their non-sleeping on request, they do not usually find the topic of sufficient interest to raise it themselves in conversation with others.

Mr K. and Mr T.

I would like to illustrate the matter further by briefly introducing two more nonsomniacs. Neither have been studied in the laboratory but they present claims which are not dissimilar from those which have been presented above. Moreover they have been kind enough to supply me with detailed reports of their sleeping and, by patiently answering strings of questions, have helped me gain a better understanding of this largely ignored phenomenon.

Mr K. is a married man, aged thirty-five, with a baby daughter. He is tall, well-built and in excellent physical health. He lives for outdoor recreation and devotes five hours of each day to organising a youth club where the emphasis is on the development of self-respect through the acquistion of skills associated with outdoor activities such as mountaineering, scuba diving, camping and sailing. During the day he works as a local government officer in a job which requires tact, sympathy and the ability to command respect. He works till 5 p.m. when he goes to the youth club. Between 10 p.m. and 12 midnight he leaves and drives home where he has his dinner. His wife retires to bed and he then sets about various hobbies which include reading, writing novels and poetry, model building and guitar playing.

His sleep report is summarised in Table 3.2. Sleep appears to be an option which was only exercised on nine out of fourteen nights and skipped when there was anything better to do. When he does sleep, he takes about one hour. On average, over the two weeks of his report he slept for 46 minutes per night, a figure similar to that computed for Miss M. He claims that he yawns a great deal during the night but never actually feels the urge to go to sleep. He does not feel that his habits are abnormal. On the contrary, he believes that others sleep for longer than they really need to.

Mr K. has had the same sleeping habits since being a young boy. His daughter appears to have inherited his nonsomnia. A baby who sleeps for only a few hours each day can create many problems for a mother who sleeps for a normal eight hours. Under such circumstances it is clearly an advantage to have a father who can go for many nights in succession without sleep! Nevertheless, my sympathy goes out to Mrs K. who must often feel thoroughly outpaced by her family.

The possibility that nonsomnia is passed on genetically is now established by a few cases. We heard from Mr H. in Perth, Australia, whose father shared nonsomnia with his son. The caller on the BBC Radio Newcastle claimed to share it with his mother and now Mr K. has a baby daughter who also sleeps very little. However, this is not the only way in which a reduction in sleep need can arise. Señora Palomino switched to non-sleeping suddenly, thirty years ago, after a painful incident involving dislocation of her jaw while yawning. Miss M. has been nonsomniac since childhood but she knows of no other example in her family nor of any relevant accounts concerning her parents. Finally, there is the extraordinary account of Mr T. who switched slowly during adolescence from being an excessive sleeper to a nonsomniac who by his own report (Table 3.3) appears to average less than 10 minutes per night.

As a young boy, Mr T. slept so well and for so long that he was very often late for school as a consequence. It was such a nuisance that he very rarely managed to get any breakfast before leaving the house each morning. This eventually became a habit which persists to this day despite his current lack of sleep. Between the ages of thirteen and sixteen the pattern changed to one where he slept for only three hours each night. This was, of course, a great

Table 3 Sleep report volunteered by Mr K.

Day of week	Fell asleep - woke up	Comments
MONDAY	NO SLEEP	4th day without sleep
TUESDAY	4.20 - 5.22 a.m. (62 min.)	Had a good sleep! Writing
WEDNESDAY	3.00 - 3.20 a.m. (20 min.)	Had a heavy day. Wrote poems
THURSDAY	12.30 - 3.15 a.m. (165 min.)	Following sauna bath. Builds oscillator for boys' club morse
FRIDAY	NO SLEEP	Driving all night to mountains
SATURDAY	1.30 - 2.25 a.m. (55 min.)	Evening spent in pub, slept soundly - camping
SUNDAY	2.10 - 3.15 a.m. (65 min.)	Hard day climbing, caught up on paperwork for club
MONDAY	NO SLEEP	Very restless after exciting weekend
TUESDAY	3.20 - 4.00 a.m. (40 min.)	Took dog for walk
WEDNESDAY	1.45 - 3.00 a.m. (75 min.)	Boring day, very tired, woke refreshed
THURSDAY	NO SLEEP	Read book on parapsychology
FRIDAY	NO SLEEP	Spending weekend on boat
SATURDAY	? (120 min?)	No clock on board 'I guess about 2 hours sleep'
SUNDAY	1.50 - 2.35 a.m. (45 min.)	Reading and working on model boat
	Average = 46 min. per night	

convenience for a young boy who was just beginning to broaden his interests. From the age of sixteen onwards he recalls only rarely sleeping for more than fifteen minutes. It is interesting that he developed asthma at roughly the same time (Miss M. also suffers from asthma but Mr K. does not).

Like Mr K., he is well-built and physically very fit. He spends a great deal of time with children and adolescents, encouraging them to enjoy themselves through outdoor activities. He was formerly a mountain rescue instructor and benefited greatly from his ability to stay awake for very long periods without strain during rescue operations. He is very much involved in the life of the community and his job requires that he be 'on call' at all hours of the night to deal with emergencies involving a large group of adolescent children for whom he is responsible. Mr T. is unmarried and reports no other incidence of nonsomnia in his immediate family.

Table 3.3 Sleep report volunteered by Mr T.

Day of week	Fell asleep - woke up	Comments
MONDAY	NO SLEEP	Music, reading, planning
TUESDAY	NO SLEEP	Travelling
WEDNESDAY	3.00 - 3.30 a.m. (30 min.)	Entertaining till late
THURSDAY	?	
FRIDAY	?	
SATURDAY	3.30 - 3.50 a.m. (20 min.)	Entertaining, music, planning
SUNDAY	2.15 - 2.18 a.m. (3 min.) 4.00 - 4.14 a.m. (14 min.)	Dreamt! Dreamt again, reading, music
MONDAY	NO SLEEP	Entertaining till late (3.00 a.m.)
TUESDAY	NO SLEEP (?)	Play cards, driving
WEDNESDAY	NO SLEEP	Planning, driving, visits homes
THURSDAY	2.00 - 2.30 a.m. (30 min.)	Driving, music, reading
FRIDAY	3.30 - 3.34 a.m. (4 min.)	Emergencies, reading
SATURDAY	NO SLEEP	Emergencies
SUNDAY	NO SLEEP	Toothache
	Average (for 12 nights) = 8.4 min.	

Two more cases

Recently, I have been given information on two more short sleepers, who have been investigated by other researchers. The first case[7] is a fifty-year-old lady who sought medical help for various reasons including her husband's concern at her abnormal habit of not sleeping. They were considering a possible link between her nonsomnia and a distressing sequence of abnormal births. Out of ten pregnancies she had produced only four normal babies. The remaining six were anencephalic, non-viable babies suffering from a serious failure of brain development.

During a short visit to hospital, the nurses were able to confirm a total absence of sleep and examination revealed some abnormal brain electrical activity (localised subcortical discharge in the left anterior Sylvian region). This suggests that the anencephalic children may have suffered from some hereditary complaint which had affected her only slightly. Her nonsomnia is a condition which has existed from childhood and her mother and sister also sleep very poorly. These facts also support the idea that her lack of sleep is an inherited condition.

There are no indications that not sleeping interfered directly with her personal or social life. No signs of sleepiness are reported and it appears that she used the night hours for housework. The reports describe her as a very active, forceful and efficient character, meticulous in appearance and involved in a wide range of social activities. There is no evidence that her nonsomnia was anything other than a symptom of an inherited condition which probably involved, in her case, only minor structural abnormalities of the brain. It was subsequently demonstrated that her sleep-control system was still largely intact since she began to sleep more normally after regular administration of tryptophan and monoamino oxidase inhibitor drugs.

Even more recently,[8] a report of short sleepers has been issued from the sleep laboratory of the Univeristy of Ottawa. Clinical researchers Roger Broughton, Donald Stuss and Thomas Healey took upon themselves the thankless task of trying to capture a few nonsomniacs for laboratory study. They found, as I did, that short sleepers are typically very busy people who attach little importance to their sleeping (or non-sleeping) habits. While they are happy to discuss their sleeping patterns with researchers, they are understandably reluctant to give up the necessary week or so of their time for the investigation of what they consider to be a relatively unimportant aspect of their make-up. This would be sacrifice enough for normal people but for the tightly scheduled and frequently overcommitted nonsomniac, it is often just too much.

Of the many people they talked to, one twenty-five-year-old man who claimed to sleep for less than two hours a day was eventually brought to bed in the laboratory. On two consecutive nights he slept for an average of 1 hour 36 minutes. Performance tests given during the observation period showed that he was not suffering from sleep deprivation at all. On a subsequent occasion his sleep was reduced to 42 minutes each night for two successive nights by the researchers. The same performance tests revealed little impairment as a consequence.

Dr Broughton tells me that this nonsomniac was a larger-than-life character who found his lack of need for sleep very useful in his chosen profession of union negotiator. His ability to remain alert and cheerful on only 30 minutes sleep per day must give him a substantial psychological advantage over antagonists in extended bargaining sessions. This stable and highly active extrovert adopted this sleep pattern during the Second World War when working shifts on radar watch at all hours. He found that he was able to keep up this life-style after the war. Like other nonsomniacs he is very jealous of his time and arranges for himself a very heavy schedule each day. He is not aware of having much spare time but feels sorry for those people who miss out by having to sleep for eight hours each day!

Nonsomnia resulting from brain damage

One individual, investigated by Mme Catherine Fischer-Perroudon[9] and reported in her PhD thesis, was seriously ill with a rare form of chorea. This illness produces a large number of unpleasant symptoms which include spasms of muscle activity in the body and face, burning and pricking sensations in the hands and feet, pruritis, sweating crises, fast heartbeat and an abnormally high temperature. The sleep of this patient was normal before the onset of the illness but subsequently he experienced little or no pressure to sleep. For four months he lived with no sleep at all without any signs of sleepiness or impaired intellectual functioning during the day. At night he often hallucinated and expressed a strong desire for sleep which reflected a need to escape from the wretchedness of his condition rather than any drowsiness.

It is the opinion of the investigator that these symptoms,

including the sleeplessness, were caused by growing brain damage caused by the disease. The possibility that the lack of sleep itself caused the other symptoms is rejected as unlikely. The fact is that the sleep-control centres in the brain lie very close to other centres which influence, among other things, sweating, breathing and heartbeat. Indiscriminate damage in that area could influence a whole range of functions in parallel.

Another case of nonsomnia, resulting from accidental brain damage, has recently been studied in Paris.[10] On this occasion a young man was involved in a serious automobile accident which rendered him comatose for one month and resulted in considerable brain damage. In the year which followed he made a remarkable recovery and now lives an almost normal life in a foreign country with a young wife whom he married after the accident. Before his accident he slept normally but now requires only four hours sleep per night - a claim which was substantiated by sleep laboratory investigations. The nonsomnia was not a matter of concern to the man but he sought advice as the result of pressure from his wife who felt that it was abnormal. Despite the reduction in sleeping time, the patient reports no sleepiness during the day and finds that it does not interfere with his effectiveness at all. It is his wife, not himself, who suffers from his lack of sleep!

Summary

We have looked for and found a number of instances, among men and other animals, where the amount of time spent sleeping is substantially lower than restorative theories of the purpose of sleep would lead us to expect. Such evidence is clearly in support of the notion that the major function of sleep is to immobilise man and animals for tactical reasons. It also suggests that any recuperation which does take place during the sleeping period could just as well happen during periods of quiet rest. In other words, the evidence appears to run contrary to the idea that sleep exists to permit certain vital physiological repair processes which can only take place at that time.

I admit that the case would be more conclusive if we were able to find and authenticate a total nonsomniac who, after many years of non-sleeping, remained a healthy, happy and effective individual. It is my firm opinion that it will not be long before this occurs. In addition we might hope that, in the not too distant future, physiologists will acquire enough detailed knowledge of the physiology of sleep control mechanisms for then to be able to disable the system by brain lesion or by chemical injection, thus producing a totally nonsomniac animal which was otherwise healthy and normal.

Observations of human nonsomniacs indicate that reduced sleep need can either be inherited or acquired. If it is acquired then our best hunch is that some change of brain functioning has occurred either through accidental brain damage, pressure on certain nerves or through some kind of poorly understood form of biochemical disturbance. It is unlikely that people can become nonsomniac by effort of will although it appears to be fairly easy to reduce one's sleeping time by an hour or so. Long sleepers who want to reap the benefits of nonsomnia may need to wait for the results of the patient and painstaking efforts of the biochemist. My hunch is that the wait need not be too long.

4 Sleep deprivation

The nonsomniacs whom we met in chapter 3 seem to have little difficulty in staying awake for long periods without harm, but this is not true for everyone. Such is the force of the pressure to sleep that few of us ever stay awake for more than a single night in a whole lifetime. Under laboratory conditions, where there is constant supervision and encouragement, a period of four days without sleep is considered to be a severe deprivation. Only seven men have sustained more than eight days of sleeplessness under scientific scrutiny and only one man has managed it for more than ten days. What then are the effects of sleep deprivation and why is it so difficult to stay awake?

Public interest in this research has unfortunately been focused almost exclusively on the more dramatic reports of visual hallucinations and other symptoms resembling mental breakdown and this may have led to a number of misconceptions. It is true that hallucinations have sometimes occurred, although some of these were merely misperceptions such as voices or distorted images. Some indeed were full blown hallucinations with psychotic qualities. One man saw a gorilla appear in the corner of the room and move threateningly towards him. The vision was so real that he ran out of the room; at which point the hallucination ceased. Nevertheless, we must not draw far-reaching conclusions without a pause for thought.

These bizarre events are somewhat exceptional occurrences. For every man who suffers a temporary breakdown under severe sleep deprivation conditions, there are many more who experience only nausea and extreme fatigue. There is certainly no guarantee that sleep deprivation of willing volunteers will produce psychotic symptoms. Many sleep experts are of the opinion that such effects are only made manifest in candidates who, in any case, have had unusual personalities and abnormal personal histories.[1]

More common are the mild changes in thinking and attitude which suggest that the sleep-deprived man is much less in contact with reality. He often does not seem to care to think straight and is less critical of his misperceptions. He often lets his imagination take over and he allows himself to think things which are simply not true. Irritability can increase and he may even be ready to believe that his experimenters are torturers. His motivation to continue becomes gradually weaker with the result that he needs more and more encouragement to stay awake.

From the subjective point of view, sleep deprivation leads to overwhelming tiredness and an intense desire to sleep. The nausea which we feel arises from our continued efforts to resist and stay awake. It is impossible to be witty, relaxed and urbane when every minute we are fighting against our own deepest wishes. Quite soon in sleep-deprivation experiments, volunteers develop a sense of the futility of the whole exercise and they would readily give it up if it were not for the encouragement of others who are not themselves tired.

Testing the effects of sleep deprivations

Psychologists have attempted to assess the effects of sleep deprivation objectively using batteries of standard tests only to discover that it is not very easy. Ian Oswald,[2] one of the first experimenters in this field, describes how

> psychologists were nonplussed by the apparent lack of any effects of sleep loss on the tasks they gave to volunteers. After three days and nights without sleep the grip was as strong as before, so evidently the muscles were not fatigued. After a request to add up a list of sums, arithmetical performance seemed no worse and no better than before, so evidently the brain could still work as cleverly. Asked to respond as quickly as possible by pressing a key after a light flash which was preceded by a warning buzzer, reaction-time could be as quick as ever.

It has been assumed that sleep deprivation resulted in muscle fatigue and the impairment of the psychological faculties of perception, memory and reasoning. This expectation was based on the idea that sleep was necessary to counteract 'brain-fatigue'. A host of experiments have shown however that the brain is capable of functioning normally in many respects even after three or four days of deprivation. The real effects of sleeplessness turn out to be somewhat more indirect.

Some tests have been devised which are sensitive to lack of sleep. These are typically monotonous and time-consuming. For example a sleep-deprived man can add two numbers together with no special difficulty. If he is asked to repeat this simple task one hundred times he will begin to make many mistakes which he would not otherwise make. Similarly, a tired man can often drive a motor car very effectively across town in heavy traffic but have great difficulty in driving for long periods along the motorway.

The problem appears to be one of concentration. Sleep deprivation undermines our ability to maintain concentration on a task which we could otherwise carry out quite well. This effect is quite marked for boring tasks but may be absent if the task is important or interesting. Wilkinson, of the Applied Psychology Research Unit in Cambridge, is one of the world's experts at producing monotonous tests for sleep-deprived naval ratings to do. These last from fifteen minutes to an hour and may involve hundreds of simple additions or listening through earphones for a quiet signal which occurs only rarely against a background of cackle. It is difficult to maintain concentration on these tests at the best of times but they are especially difficult to do when sleep deprived. By contrast, he once devised an intellectually challenging battle-game. His sleep-deprived naval ratings were able to play this game for over an hour without showing any impairment due to their ordeal. The interest of the game was enough to help maintain their concentration.

Experiments of this kind make it clear that sleep deprivation does not interfere directly with our ability to see, hear, think, remember or act. It does affect our performance by reducing our ability to concentrate on a task. As a consequence our mind wanders easily from the matter in hand causing us to make errors and to fail to notice that we are doing the wrong thing. Concentration depends upon motivation. If something is important enough or very interesting then we have little trouble in giving it our full attention. On the other hand if a task does not capture our interest then after a few minutes our attention wanders and mistakes are easily made. Sleep deprivation works by lowering our motivation and, as a consequence, our ability to concentrate is impaired.

Motivation does not disappear completely, it is merely reduced. It can still be revived by an exciting game or the arrival of a friend whose company is much enjoyed. An emergency can also shake a sleep-deprived soldier from his lethargy. The main difference is that events need to be even more stimulating than usual if they are to maintain attention for more than a few minutes. The more sleep-deprived the individual, the more quickly his motivation sags.

It is helpful to think of sleep need as a motive itself which competes with other urges and desires. Figure 4.1 illustrates this competition which can be seen in action on any normal evening. Sleep pressure rises slowly in the late evening until it is eventually more powerful than other drives. As a result we go to bed early when nothing of interest is happening but we stay up late if there is anything we badly want to do.

Sleep may fall into the special class of avoidance motives, since it involves a withdrawal from the normal scene of action to a safe place. This helps us understand our reaction to boredom. Normally we will avoid boring situations if at all possible. When this is not possible, the symptoms of sleep will appear immediately, as if by magic. It is a regrettably frequent occurrence in the life of a teacher to be faced with a class full of captive students many of whom are yawning and having difficulty staying awake. They are not sleep deprived. The desire to close their eyes and fall asleep is simply an avoidance reaction; the only one available at the time.

Aggression and fear are two other motives which occur in situations calling for avoidance. This helps us understand how sleep deprivation on the one hand causes an increase in irritability and on the other hand a tendency to exaggerate irrational fears. This results from a general mobilisation of avoidance motivation. For example, many of the hallucinations reported by researchers take the form of threatening spectres rather than beatific visions. Rare cases of psychotic behaviour, during sleep deprivation stress,

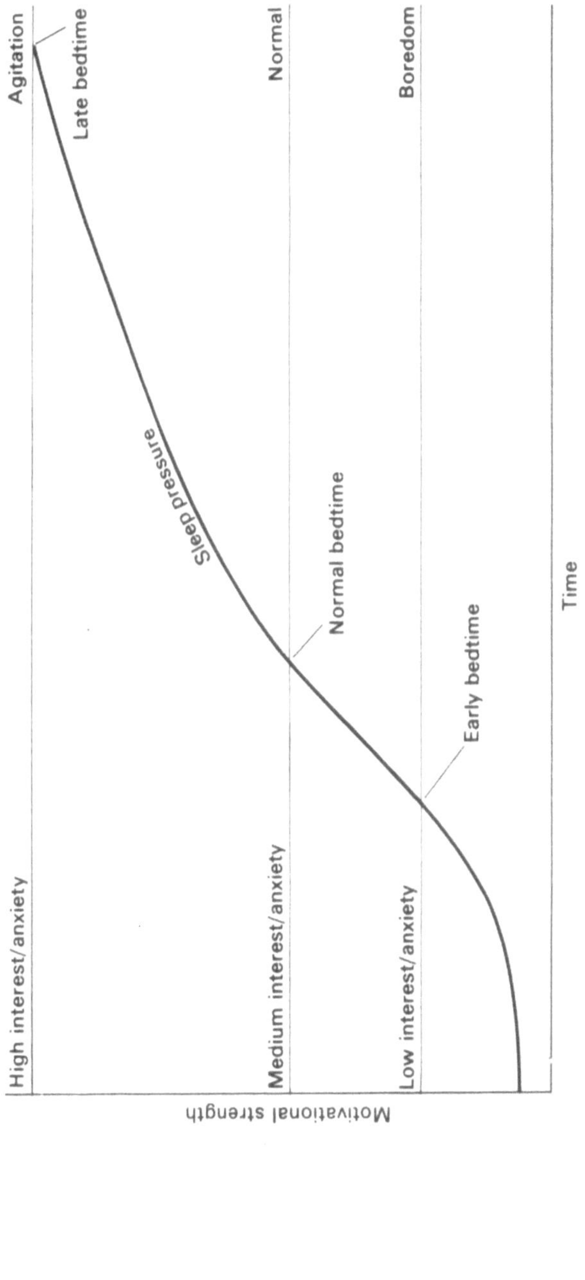

Figure 4.1 Choice of bedtime results from a competition between rising sleep pressure and other motives

often involve a paranoid mixture of fear and aggression. Peter West, the disc jockey who stayed awake for 200 hours as a publicity stunt, produced these symptoms towards the end of his vigil which manifested themselves in the belief that others were trying to undermine his efforts by secretly drugging him.

Sleep may combine with other avoidance motives according to the situation. When nothing can be done to avoid pain, as in the boring lecture, the desire to be free from the situation intensifies sleepiness. On the other hand if aversive action is possible sleep may be supressed. This occurs in emergencies when sleepiness is usually reduced. Webb compared two methods of keeping rats awake and found that electric shocks were much less successful than non-punitive, positive stimulation such as handling and feeding them. Using electric shock, he found extreme sleepiness after only thirty hours while non-punitive treatment revealed no signs of sleepiness even after four days.

This perspective gives us some insight into the use of sleep deprivation as a torture. Brutal treatment in captive conditions may accentuate the sleep drive. If the brutality is also apparently the result of dozing then the prisoner is caught up in a vicious circle of pain and helplessness where he appears to be inflicting pain upon himself by falling asleep. The effectiveness of this treatment, when it is effective, probably derives mainly from the prisoner's sense of helplessness.

Sleep deprivation and the need for recovery

In a recent review, by my colleague Jim Horne[3] of the biochemical and psychophysiological effects of total sleep deprivation, very few reliable physiological effects were found. He concluded that 'the major effects of sleep deprivation lie with behaviour and performance, that is within the brain rather than the body'. This view is very encouraging to the sleep instinct concept which considers sleep need to be a motivational state rather than a bodily deficit. Nevertheless, many people believe that the behavioural changes observed after sleep loss result from some accumulated deficit in the brain. This theory implies that sleep is necessary to permit certain vital processes (physiological or intellectual), which cannot take place when awake. If we do not sleep then these processes do not take place and we suffer accordingly.

There is no doubt that we do suffer when sleep deprived. Whether or not we suffer because of the lack of these vital recovery processes is another question which we shall now consider. The problem is not made easy by the failure of recuperation theorists to specify precisely what these processes are. Hartmann,[4] in his recent statements on the functions of sleep, illustrates this point very well. He suggests that slow wave sleep '*could* be a phase when macromolecules - protein *and/or* RNA - are synthesised, especially in the central nervous system' (my italics). He is of necessity silent on the matter of *which* macromolecules are involved and he says little to explain why we need to be unconscious to synthesise them when we know that protein manufacture can take place at all times. Moreover, Hartmann himself would be the first to admit that even this vague statement goes far beyond the available evidence. Of course the failure to specify which recuperative processes are involved does not necessarily prove that there aren't any: it could be seen as merely illustrating how elusive they are.

The sleep deprivation experiments do, however, show another important effect which is consistent with the idea of repair and recovery. This is the *rebound effect.* If you miss sleep on one night, you make it up by sleeping more on the next night. It is as if your body 'knows' just how much sleep it needs and has some special system for making sure that it gets its quota. Unfortunately, we are again faced with an ambiguity which makes this argument seem a little unconvincing. The amount of 'recovery' sleep does not correspond with the amount of sleep lost. After many days of sleep deprivation complete recovery is usually experienced after four to eight hours of extra sleep, just a fraction of the twenty to forty hours that he may have lost. It is possible that the repair process is speeded up in such an emergency but once again it would be necessary to know something about these mysterious processes before a proper assessment could be made of this suggestion. Sleep-deprivation experiments do certainly produce results which are suggestive of some recovery process but it is not yet certain that the sleeper, during rebound, is really recovering from the lack of some repair process which he has missed.

An alternative explanation

The concept of 'pressure to sleep' is an important part of the immobilisation hypothesis (the theory that we sleep to keep out of trouble), and it will prove even more useful in helping us to understand the effects of sleep deprivation without recourse to any mysterious recovery processes. Sleep pressure is an integral part of the sleep instinct mechanism whose aim is to cause an animal to give up whatever it is doing and to go find a suitable sleep site. Sleep pressure works by undermining our motivation to continue with any activity. If we are engaged in a relatively unimportant and tedious task then sleep pressure, in the form of drowsiness, will cause us to give it up readily. If it is more important, or more interesting, then we will usually persist with the task until the sleep pressure becomes stronger.

Concentration is affected most because it represents our motivation to attend. We have difficulty in concentrating on a boring lecture because we are not motivated to attend. Because sleep pressure undermines our motivation, it automatically spoils our ability to concentrate. If our motivation is improved by some emergency or novelty then concentration can be readily, however temporarily, restored. The art of keeping people awake during sleep-deprivation experiments involves keeping the volunteers' motivation high in one way or another.

The sleep instinct has a fail-safe device whereby the animal or person cannot fall asleep when he is engaged in motivated behaviour. The reason for this is obvious, but it does mean that the sleep-pressure mechanism should have some way of bringing this behaviour to an orderly conclusion. Otherwise we might never get to bed. It does this by slowly and delicately nibbling away at the motivational systems so that we lose interest in what we are doing. When the sleep instinct finally succeeds and the animal is lying snugly in a safe place with its thoughts drifting gently about, then, and only then, can sleep move in and take over.

We can now see that sleep-deprived man will obviously experience difficulties in concentration which will become even more acute as time passes. This is because the pressure to sleep is being slowly but relentlessly increased. Because his motivation has been reduced, he is less willing to expend much energy and his attention wanders easily when he is forced to do a boring job. Moreover, he requires more and more incentive to continue with the experiment which appears increasingly futile and pointless. At the same time he is suffering from sore eyes and muscular irritation which, as we have already seen, are used as incentives to make sleep an attractive proposition. Finally, he will be suffering from the fatigue produced by the additional muscular activity which is always required to keep sleep at bay.

Hallucinations

This account brings us a little nearer to an explanation of defects of attention and performance but does not immediately account for the misperceptions or even the hallucinations which are occasionally reported. These only occur after prolonged deprivation when the volunteer subjects are under very considerable pressure to fall asleep. At these times we might expect that the subjects will indeed dip briefly into light stages of sleep during unoccupied moments and it is quite possible that the imaginative misperceptions of sleep-deprived subjects occur at these times. Oswald[5] puts it thus: 'Just as visions are common when falling asleep in bed, in the same way, a sleep-deprived man, forced to walk about with his eyes open, often describes "seeing things".'

Unfortunately, very few sleep researchers have turned their scientific attention to the visions which sometimes occur as normal people begin to fall asleep, known as hypnagogic phenomena. Fortunately anecdotal evidence abounds and there are many stories of sounds such as voices calling one's name or loud bangs, light flashes as well as flashes of pseudo-poetic inspiration. I have never experienced them myself and therefore stand at a disadvantage when discussing the matter. But I am assured that these experiences carry with them the conviction of reality such that the sleeper may sit up with a start and be sure that he 'heard something'. This sense of reality is in good agreement with the reports of the sleep-deprived people who describe brief misperceptions.

In an attempt to become privy to these hypnagogic secrets, I have, on a number of occasions, allowed myself to fall asleep under controlled conditions in my own sleep laboratory. I retire to bed with electrodes fixed to my head and face while an assistant watches the indications of my brainwave activity on the polygraph. He can see when the first signs of sleep appear. Then, after a minute of sleep, he wakes me up and tape records an immediate account of my experience.

Alas, I have no dramatic visions to report, nor inspired sillinesses. But I can reveal a distinct change in the quality of my thoughts. Before falling asleep I am aware of a directed line of thinking as I mull over a problem such as how to sound-proof the laboratory so that the noises of my assistant no longer prevent me from falling asleep. On forced arousal I notice that my thoughts still concern the same kind of ideas – indeed I am initially tempted to deny that I was asleep – but on reflection it is evident that the thoughts were no longer under conscious control. My thinking had begun to drift around from idea to idea, merely by a process of association, an experience very similar to that of the daydream. This description compares well with other descriptions I have read. The loss of mental discipline without any loss of thought content could well be an important influence on the thinking of individuals who have suffered prolonged sleep deprivation.

None of this is sufficient to explain the vivid hallucinations which are reported by some sleep-deprived subjects. These are described by the psychiatrically trained as closely resembling psychotic delusions or the fantasies of individuals on LSD 'trips'. It is difficult to know what to make of the comparison with the psychoses since we still know so little about them. But the comparison with the effects of LSD may prove more helpful, as a result of recent research into the chemicals which are used by the brain to control sleep.

One such chemical is serotonin,[6] which has a chemical structure similar in many respects to LSD. It is believed by many researchers that serotonin accumulates during wakefulness in a large group of cells called the raphe nuclei in the brain stem, one of the older and more primitive areas of our nervous system. These cells have projections which travel long distances to many other parts of the brain. When these cells become active, as they probably do, especially during sleep, the serotonin is believed to be released from the tips of these projections causing other cells in various parts of the brain to be affected.

It is possible that this release of serotonin acts like a very mild dose of LSD which under normal circumstances causes loss of concentration and thought discipline. This is normally harmless and merely encourages us to give up what we are trying to do and to go to bed. During sleep deprivation, brief periods of sleep will result in the softening up of thought processes and encourage misperceptions. If serotonin builds up gradually in the raphe cells during wakefulness, then we might expect a sleep-deprived person to experience these break-throughs into sleep more often or, alternatively, the brief sleep episodes may be accompanied by a more copious discharge of serotonin throughout the brain which might, in turn, cause effects akin to those of a full LSD trip. Of course, the release would be terminated when the subject snaps awake again or is shaken by the experimenter. Experiments have indeed shown that subjects can shake out of their hallucinations which rarely last for very long.

The serotonin build-up theory is still controversial but I hope that by now you will agree that there is a case for treating the effects of sleep deprivation as the result of an internally triggered pressure to sleep applied by the sleep instinct. Some of the less sensational effects, such as lack of concentration or lowered motivation, are simply exaggerations of the common experience of drowsiness. The loose thinking and misperceptions as well as the bizarre hallucinations are caused by the sleep process breaking temporarily through the efforts of will of the sleep-deprived man. This explanation is simple and has the advantage that it does not need to invoke the failure of mysterious repair processes to carry out healing work. If it is the correct explanation then we may no longer regard the hallucinatory effects of sleep deprivation as critical evidence in favour of the recuperative theories of the function of sleep.

Recovery from sleep deprivation

The idea of a pressure build-up can also explain why we sleep longer after a period of sleep deprivation. The sleep instinct has been designed to begin with only gradual pressure which would not seriously interfere with anything but the most monotonous tasks. The aim of the instinct is, of course, to nudge you to go to bed rather than to cause you to fall down asleep there and then. If the call is not heeded then the pressure is built up slowly so that an effort of will of greater and greater strength is required to resist it. If the situation is an emergency, or otherwise full of interest, then the effort of will can be found; otherwise we give in and go to bed.

It is possible that this increased pressure is caused by accumulations of the chemical serotonin in raphe nuclei in the brain stem which can only be properly released during sleep. It follows that the release of this serotonin will take longer if more of it has accumulated before the sleep session begins. This will lead to a sleep rebound and extra sleep may be required to bring the pressure down to normal.

If you miss a night's sleep then we can assume that the accumulation of serotonin will be much greater by the time you go to bed next evening. This means that the inital rate of discharge of serotonin will be faster soon after going to sleep because of the increased pressure and as a result the eight hours worth of extra pressure, from the night before, may be discharged in only three extra hours or so. This increased pressure produces a law of diminishing returns so that the amount of additional recovery sleep required becomes progressively less for each additional night spent awake (Figure 4.2).

This is what we observe in the sleep laboratory, so that it is rare to hear of anyone who sleeps for more than sixteen hours even after severe loss of sleep. According to the immobilisation hypothesis this is what we might expect because the additional sleep offers very little by way of a survival advantage. For many animals a long sleep could lead to death by starvation. It is understandable that the sleep pressure mechanism could lead to an overshoot if it is stretched to unnatural lengths but it has also proved necessary in the course of evolution to devise an arrangement whereby this overshoot can be kept to a tolerable minimum.

Dream deprivation

So far I have confined my attention to the effects of total sleep deprivation and have attempted to show that these are compatible

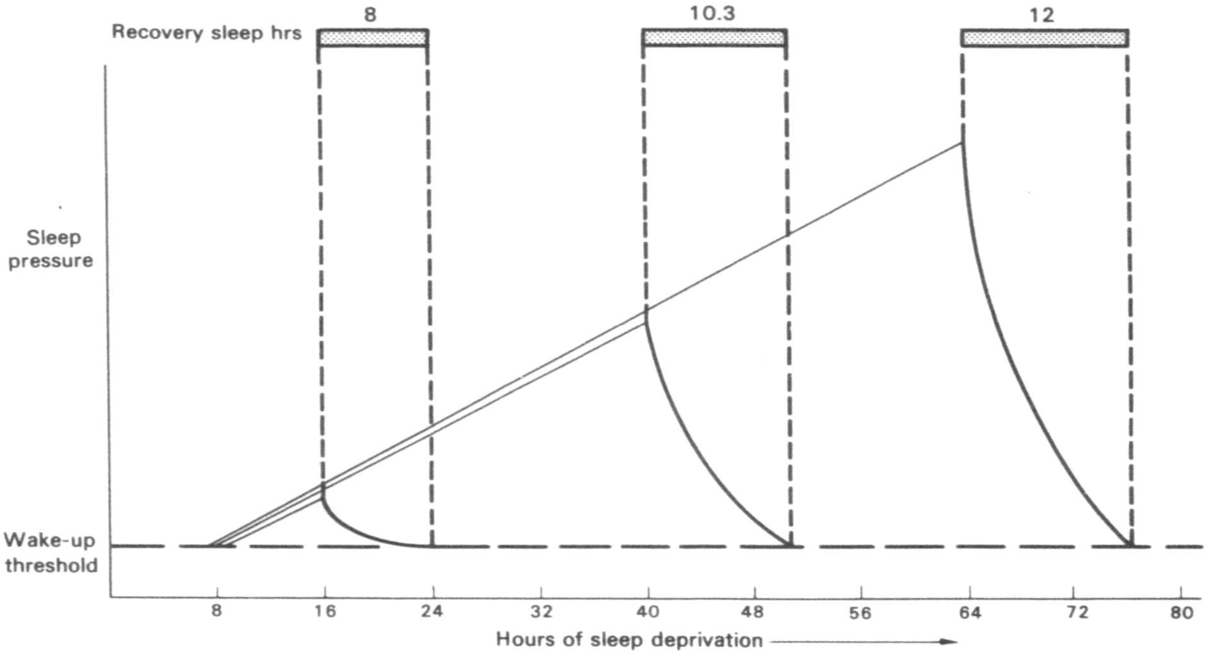

Figure 4.2 Increase in sleeping time following sleep deprivation is only modest; this would follow if the increase in sleep pressure (during waking) is linear while the decrease (during sleep) is exponential

with the theory that the instinct to sleep serves some simple purpose such as the need to keep out of trouble. I have also tried to show that deprivation studies do not particularly favour recuperative theories rather than more simple sleep instinct theories. In doing so I have ignored the 'dream deprivation' studies which many theorists set great store by. My reason for ignoring them has been simply that I expect total-sleep-deprivation studies to be a more effective technique than selective studies, for providing a basis for a discussion as to whether sleep serves *any* repair function. My conclusion is that the evidence is not very strong on this point. As a result I do not expect selective deprivation studies to be any more helpful.

Nevertheless, I realise that they cannot be dismissed so lightly, and some discussion will clearly be required. Much of the interest in this aspect of sleep research was caused by a widely discussed early report by Dement,[7] an eminent pioneer of sleep research. His experiments appeared to show that if people were deprived of the kind of sleep which accompanies dreams two dramatic effects occurred. First, the subjects of his experiments would subsequently spend more time in this kind of sleep as if catching up on a need. Second, it seemed that this treatment might precipitate psychosis in the deprived volunteers. The myth that dream deprivation leads to madness was born.

The simple truth is that madness is not caused by this treatment. None of the many experiments which have since tested this idea have shown any signs of madness whatsover. Dement has himself expressed public misgivings about the original experiment and has even stated categorically that 'no study has shown that REM (dream) deprivation has significant functional consequences for the waking life of human subjects.'[8] But the myth lives on.

Certain types of antidepressant drugs have the effect of suppressing dreaming sleep entirely. Clinical cases have been reported which describe patients who have gone for many months without any dreaming sleep at all as the result of taking these drugs. During this time the patient shows a distinct improvement of mood and ability to cope with problems. Dream deprivation may have even helped them recover.

Vogel,[9] a clinician at the Georgia Mental Health Institute in the USA, is even using dream deprivation as a technique for curing depression and claims to have had considerable success. The patient sleeps in the laboratory for six consecutive nights and is prevented from dreaming by a forced arousal whenever the recording machine indicates that a dream is imminent. The reduction in depressive symptoms which they observe lends support to the idea that antidepressant drugs cure depression partly by their ability to suppress dreaming sleep.

These results agree in general terms with the animal experiments which often involve very prolonged dream deprivation lasting up to thirty days. Dement reports that 'no consistent changes were observed in the basic perceptual and motor functions and there was no evidence of a disruption or impairment in high level processes, such as learning and memory.'[10] The changes which were observed could be described as an enhancement of drive motivation, such as an increase in aggressiveness or sexual behaviour. Since the alleviation of depression may reasonably be described in terms of an enhanced motivational state, the animal and human studies appear to be in happy agreement. Not only does dream deprivation not lead to madness, it may even be useful as a cure for it in certain cases!

There is no controversy about the rebound phenomenon. This is well attested by many experiments, but it would be foolish to fall into the trap of thinking that a rebound indicates a need for dreaming sleep in the sense that certain vital intellectual functions occur while dreaming (functions which we cannot do without). It would be foolish to believe this because we have already seen that people can do without it and that some people may even be better off without it. The system appears to work by the build-up of biochemical pressures and is liable to small overshooting if normal functioning is disturbed. Let us be clear that the overshoot after dream deprivation is always very small compared with the amount of dreaming sleep which has been lost. For example, after ten nights without dreams the extra dreaming sleep on the 'recovery' night is rarely more than that lost on a single night.[11]

The idea that we need to sleep in order to dream is now a dead duck, but we can be sure that it will not lie down. It is a romantic notion that dreams work for you during the night; a notion which appeals to us all. But if scientific evidence is needed to shore up this poetic hypothesis, the world of sleep research is currently in no position to oblige. Our willingness to adhere to the notion is probably due in part to the time-honoured view, taught in childhood, that sleep heals and repairs our weary bodies and minds. Early sleep research seemed to be offering clues as to how this healing process works, but the tide has turned and the early promise has faded.

The main problem is that both the restoration theory and the immobilisation theory agree that there exists a powerful mechanism inside both man and animals whose function is to cause us to go to sleep reliably often and in an orderly fashion. There is no dispute about this. The effects of sleep-deprivation experiments, whether formal or informal, give us an appreciation of just how difficult it is to resist this mechanism but they do not give us any clue as to why the mechanism should be there in the first place or as to what purpose sleep serves. Such experiments do give us insight into how the sleep instinct manages to win every time, no matter how strong the opposition, but this insight is not enough to help us decide whether the purpose of sleep is one of behavioural strategy or physiological recovery. Traditionally, the effects of sleep deprivation have been quoted as the strongest evidence in favour of recuperation theories. On closer inspection, this turns out to be unjustified, and alternative interpretations of the data are possible. It now seems that the major supporting argument in favour of recuperation theories is no longer valid. Perhaps the time has come to abandon such notions altogether.

5 Dreaming sleep

Many people believe that we need to sleep in order to dream and that we need to dream in order either to resolve our emotional conflicts, or solve our intellectual problems, or release surplus instinctual energy, or rearrange our untidy information stores, or consolidate new memories. Take any one or any combination or permutation of these possible functions and you have a ready-made, modern theory of the function of dreams which will at least please some of the people some of the time.

These theories received a terrific boost when it was discovered by sleep researchers that dreams typically occur at specific times during sleep, when the eyes of the sleeper could be seen to dart back and forth under closed eye-lids. These rapid-eye-movement (REM) periods occupied about one and a half hours of our total sleep time of eight hours.[1] Dreams had finally arrived in the sterile world of the hard-nosed sleep researcher and the evidence seemed to indicate that they were important. Why else would they occupy such a large proportion of the night? Why else would dreaming time increase following experiments when volunteers had been dream deprived?

The biggest boost came when reports appeared which suggested that dream-deprived people showed psychotic symptoms. These early experiments are still quoted widely in popular articles on the meaning of dreams. Unfortunately it has not proved possible to repeat this finding and, as we saw in chapter 4, the evidence no longer supports the need-for-dreams theory in this particular respect and few serious sleep researchers now believe that dream-deprivation does any harm at all. We also saw in chapter 4 that some procedures for treating depression actually involve depriving patients of their dreams, either by using drugs or by waking patients whenever a dream period begins.

Some findings do still stand, however. Dream-deprived people show an increase in dreaming time when they are allowed to sleep normally, although this is usually a small and diminishing proportion of the total amount of lost dream time. Nevertheless, the major piece of evidence, supporting the basic idea that dreams are necessary for sanity, has now gone and dream-repair theories remain as much a matter of faith as they always have been.

There is no denying that good things may indeed happen to us during dreams, such as memory reorganisation. What is in question is whether these good things are essential to our physical and mental health or even to the survival of our species. We know that the dream control mechanism is an elaborate one. Was it built over millions of years of evolutionary history simply to give us healing fantasies or was its existence called into being by other more prosaic factors?

Any good general theory of sleep must supply a satisfactory answer to this question. So far, the immobilisation theory of sleep has been quite silent on this issue. After all, if sleep merely serves to keep animals out of trouble, why should sleep need to be so complex? Why do we need two types of sleep, dreaming and non-dreaming sleep? Early versions of the theory ignored dreaming sleep and admitted this as a weakness but recently it has been possible to piece together new evidence to produce a possible theory. It is still a very new theory and therefore very open to discussion. For an informed argument we shall need to know some facts. Accordingly I shall review some of the most important facts now, and later (in chapter 6) argue the case for the new theory.

What is dreaming sleep?

The modern scientific concept of dreaming sleep began with the discovery of rapid-eye-movement (REM) periods which occurred at intervals throughout the night. Volunteers, when woken from REM sleep, frequently reported that they had been dreaming and would often be able to give a vivid account of their dream on request. It was also discovered that the electrical rhythms of the brain resembled those of wakefulness during REM episodes while during non-dreaming sleep the electrical rhythms were characteristically different having more in common with the brain rhythms of comatose patients. The actual patterns need not concern us. The main discovery was that brain activity during REM sleep was different from that of non-REM sleep but similar to that of wakefulness.

Following this discovery, many investigators looked at other aspects of bodily functioning and found, among other things, that heart beat and breathing were surprisingly irregular during REM sleep and that blood flow to the brain was increased. Casual observation of the cat or dog on your own hearthrug will show many twitches of the paws, ears and whiskers at this time. Cats and dogs also show a very deep relaxation of their main posture muscles during REM episodes which gives the animal a characteristic flat-out, floppy appearance. One of the most challenging observations concerns the erection of the penis which also takes place. In women an increase of the blood flow to genital areas has also been found. These changes are not, as one might expect, associated with erotic dreams. In any case, such dreams are really quite rare.

These changes are highly reliable and form the basis of the belief among many scientists that REM sleep is a quite different state from non-REM sleep. In a nutshell, sleep is composed of two alternating but quite distinctly different states. Among adults, and this also applies to animals, the sleep period invariably begins with a long period of non-REM sleep which is followed by a period of REM sleep. The two states alternate throughout the night in the manner shown in Figure 5.1. Human sleepers tend to have longer REM periods later in the night.

The intervals between the beginning of successive REM episodes is fairly constant at approximately 90 minutes. Among animals the switching back and forth varies from species to species. In general the rule is: the heavier the animal, the longer the interval between REM episodes. Figure 5.2 illustrates this rule. The principle has not gone uncontested by investigators[2] but is still a useful rule of thumb for animals whose sleep patterns are not interrupted by frequent and long periods of waking.

Dreams and dreaming sleep

The early studies of REM sleep showed impressive evidence for a

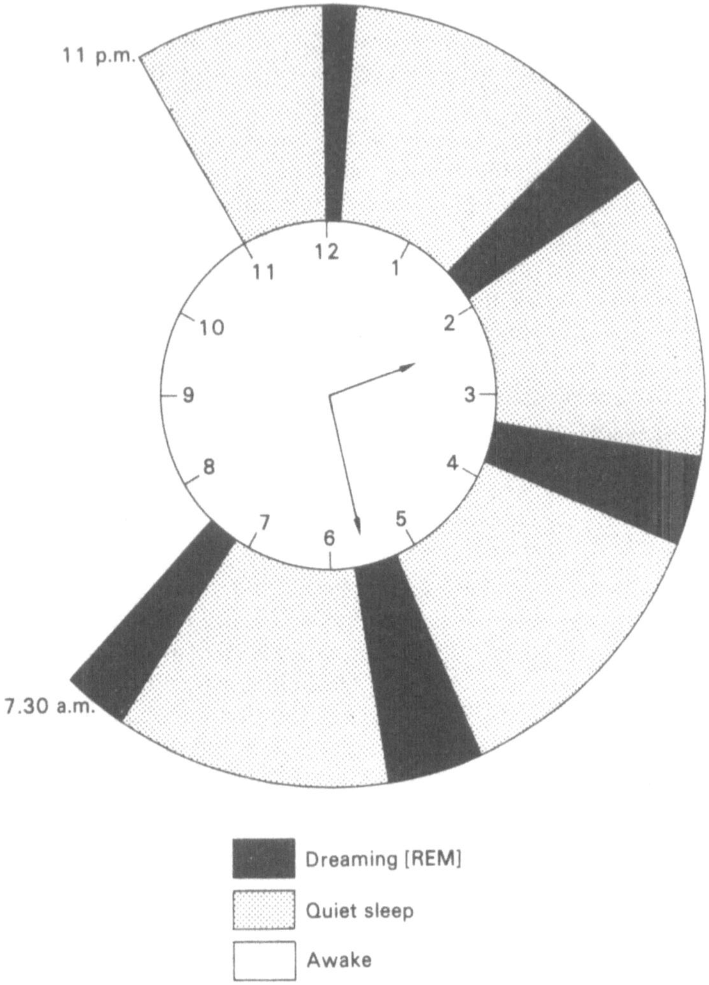

Figure 5.1 The sleep/dream cycle for a normal human adult

link between it and dreams. Much of this has had to be qualified by later analysis but the basic idea is still valid, the idea that people will often report a dream when woken from a REM episode. What is even more impressive is the fact that the length of the dream report is roughly related to the length of time spent

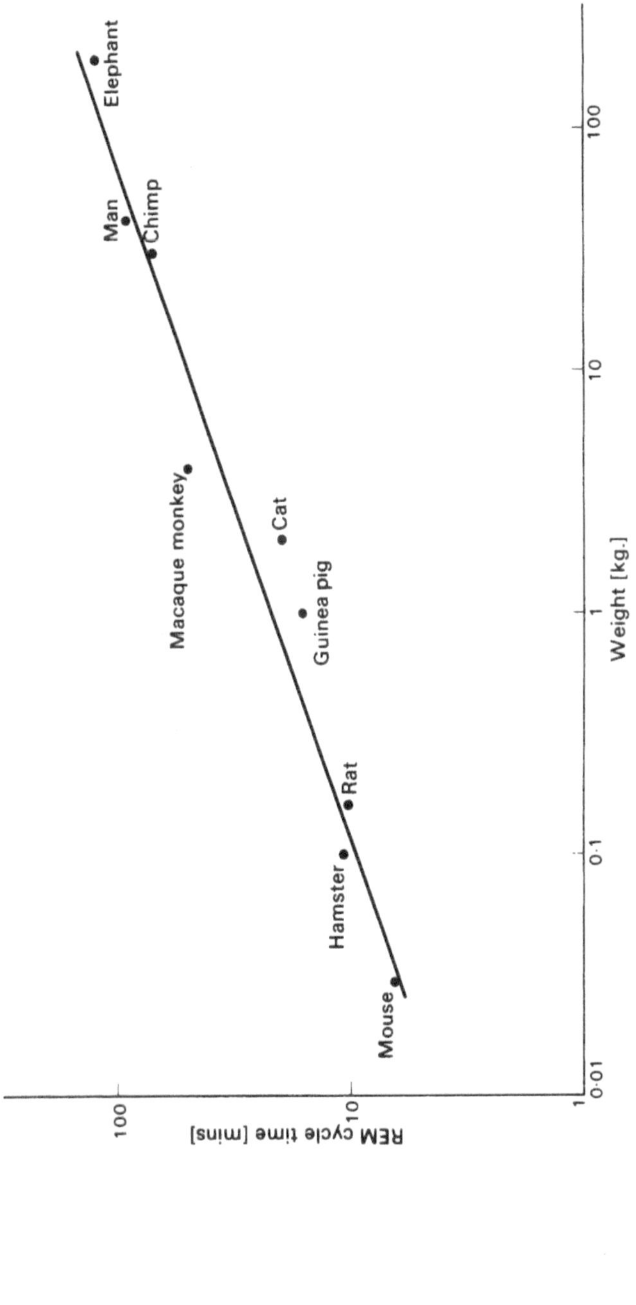

Figure 5.2 REM cycle length is correlated with weight among mammals. Log scales have been used on both axes

in REM sleep immediately before being woken up. A long spell in REM sleep typically results in a long dream narrative with lots of detail. It is clear from these results that dreams are not instantaneous, as some believed, but develop along a more natural 'thinking' time scale during the dream period.

Some early investigations seemed to show a link between the pictures of the dream and the particular eye-movements observed. This seems wholly reasonable whether you believe that the eye-movements dictate the dream content or that the dream influences the directions and frequency of the movements. These reports were met with scepticism in many quarters, however, and not all experimenters have been able to confirm these findings. The issue remains controversial and, whilst the problem is intriguing, failure to resolve it probably does not matter too much.

However impressive the link between REM sleep and dreaming, we must not adopt too simple-minded a view of the situation. For example, not all awakenings from REM sleep produce a dream report. Sometimes volunteers say that they think they were dreaming but can't remember anything specific. Sometimes they simply deny completely any awareness of dreaming. It is possible that they have simply forgotten, but this must remain only an hypothesis for the time being.

In addition we must note that dream reports can occur after arousals from non-REM sleep. This news came as something of a disappointment to the sleep-research community but careful analysis of the dream reports has shown a broad pattern of differences between those obtained following REM and non-REM sleep. REM sleep reports are more vivid, more bizarre and contain a much more obvious narrative element. Non-REM sleep reports are more of the 'thinking' variety with little vividness and less of a story like character. Nevertheless, there is considerable overlap in the quality of the actual reports and this must give us pause.

The following three examples illustrate our difficulties. These were taken from a student project carried out by Clare Bradley in my old laboratory at Bedford College, London University. Clare woke her volunteers by playing a loud rushing noise (white noise) over a loudspeaker in their bedroom. This dream report followed an arousal from non-REM sleep (i.e. so-called 'non-dreaming' sleep).

> I was dreaming all right. There was a rushing wind. I was out in the open. It was a bit of a shock when I realised that it was the sound that I had to respond to rather than what I was thinking about. I was doing something outside. I might have been digging in the garden. I can't remember any more.

Compare that with the next report which followed an awakening from clear REM sleep:

> I was on an adventure playground which I'd been to and there were some children very high up on some ropes in a tree and some kind of inspector came along and said that the tree was unsafe because it was rotten inside. He'd told them before and they hadn't taken any notice.

There is clearly more action in the second report than the first but we need to bend our definition of 'dreaming' quite a bit if we want to rule out the first report (following non-dreaming sleep!) from being classed as a 'dream'.

The third example is a report following an awakening from REM (dreaming) sleep, one hour after the last report.

> Experimenter: Were you dreaming?
> Volunteer: I think that there was something about paying back-rent or something like that. It was very vague.
> Experimenter: Can you remember anything more about it?
> Volunteer: Not really it was more – kind of – words than images.

This is the kind of report which we might have expected from non-REM sleep and it illustrates the difficulty in offering hard and fast rules concerning what constitutes dreaming and what merely constitutes thinking. It shows clearly that non-REM and REM sleep states often show overlap in the mental events which accompany them.

It is certain that mental activity of various degrees of narrative interest and clarity occurs during both REM and non-REM sleep. More lively accounts are, however, more likely to follow awakenings from REM sleep. My own view is that this change in the intensity of the mental activity is a simple, and possibly trivial, consequence of the increase in the activity of the brain which takes place during REM sleep. I do not deny that dreams are interesting in their own right. Nevertheless, I cannot believe that they tell us very much about the purpose of REM sleep. Mental activity is present all through sleep. All that happens during REM sleep is that this mental activity gets a boost and becomes a little more interesting to our waking selves, should we later remember it. Beyond that, dreaming probably has no further relevance to our understanding of the nature and function of REM sleep states.

Animal studies

Interest in the content of REM dream reports has waned considerably with the finding that almost all mammals and birds studied in the laboratory also show similar sleep states to those of human volunteers. At the time of writing I know that the list of animals which show clear signs of the REM sleep state includes chimpanzee, baboon, macaque, rhesus monkey, goat, pig, cow, horse, sheep, rabbit, elephant, cat, bottle-nose dolphin, pilot-whale, seal, bat, guinea pig, rat, chipmunk, mouse, squirrel, hamster, mole, mole-rat, tree-shrew, desert-hedgehog, armadillo, opossum, kangaroo, phalanger, owl, burrowing owl, domestic chicken, pigeon, hawk and falcon.[3] With a list like this it is tempting to wonder what they are all dreaming about. On the other hand, if we had started off with the knowledge that REM sleep was common in animals and then thought of man simply as another animal, it is highly likely that we would have attached much less importance to the dreaming aspect of the phenomenon.

As it is, the wide distribution across birds and mammals of this two-state structure of sleep is impressive and reinforces our curiosity concerning its purpose. There must be some simple explanation which applies equally well to all of the animals involved. One clue which has occurred to many researchers as relevant is the fact that only warm-blooded animals show a sleep pattern consisting of two alternating sleep states. Reptiles, which are cold-blooded (i.e. they do not maintain a high body temperature at all times) appear to have a very simple unchanging kind of sleep state. It is therefore possible that REM sleep evolved to meet the special requirements of warm-blooded mammals and birds. This is a possibility which we shall have to consider seriously in chapter 6.

New names for old

Animal studies have also made us realise how important it is to be careful about the terms we use when discussing sleep. For example, it is clearly very dangerous to use the term *dreaming sleep* when discussing the mole, since it is difficult to be sure that the mole is, in fact, dreaming. It is possible, of course, but we must not use a scientific name which assumes a fact which has not been scientifically established. A similar problem concerns the use of the term *REM sleep* which implies that rapid-eye-movements are an important feature of the state being described. In fact, there is no reason to suppose that it is any more important than other features such as the activated pattern of brain electrical activity, relaxation of the neck muscles, penile erections, irregularity of breathing and heart-beating or any other of the more technical indications which have been suggested.

The problem is made worse by the fact that sleep is always subtly different from one species to another. Some show rapid-eye-movement bursts, some do not (e.g. the owl, which, in any case, does not move its eyes when awake). Even man, who shows a lot of eye-movement activity, may show long periods of so-called REM sleep without any eye-movements at all! Similarly, the marked relaxation of neck muscle tension during REM sleep in the cat, is often unreliable in man and absent altogether in other animals such as the tree-shrew. The only feature which is always present is the activated quality of brain rhythms which resembles closely but not exactly the pattern which is normally present during alert wakefulness. This common factor has given rise to the new but increasingly popular name *active sleep* (AS) which I shall use for the remainder of this book.

The change of name is important because it reflects a significant change of attitude among scientists in recent times. The early emphasis in sleep circles was on dreams and rapid-eye-movements and the explanations of the complex dynamic structure of sleep was sought in terms of these features. This explains in part the interest in dreams as a means of recovery from intellectual and emotional stress. More recently the emphasis has been upon the various different *states* which go to make up sleep, states which can be seen just as easily in many varieties of birds and mammals.

Table 5.1 gives the new name *active sleep* along with the many other names which it has replaced. It also gives the new name of *quiet sleep* (QS) to the other state along with a variety of other names which have been used from time to time. Quiet sleep is really more complicated than its name implies and it is sometimes useful to distinguish two sub-states *light quiet sleep (LQS)* and *deep quiet sleep (DQS),* although this distinction may only be valuable for cats and primates, including man. The initials *AS* will be used from now on to indicate what we have previously called *REM sleep. QS* replaces the old term *non-REM sleep.*

Table 5.1 New names for old in sleep research

New name	Active Sleep (AS)	Quiet Sleep (QS)
Old names	rapid-eye-movement sleep (REM sleep)	orthodox sleep
	paradoxical sleep (PS)	non-REM sleep
	rhombencephalic sleep (fast sleep)	slow wave sleep (SWS)
	dreaming sleep	telencephalic sleep (slow sleep)
		non-dreaming sleep

The fragility of active sleep

One of the most fascinating facts concerning AS involves the proportion of sleep which is occupied by AS. For example, animals such as man, cats, squirrels and moles devote more than 20 per cent of their sleep to AS whereas others such as guinea pigs, rabbits, mice, sheep, cows and certain monkeys will rarely exceed a figure of 15 per cent. Table 5.2 gives a very approximate league table which can serve as a guide. The times vary, of course, from one animal to another and results may well vary from one investigator to another. Nevertheless, the broad pattern of values is stable enough to require an explanation as long as we don't take the individual values too seriously.

An interesting suggestion has been proposed by two American sleep researchers, Allison and Van Twyver,[4] who noticed that animals who sleep securely show a lot of AS. Some animals are secure during sleep, such as the squirrel and the mole because they

Table 5.2 Amount of active sleep time for various mammalian species expressed in terms of number of hours per day (see chapter 2, note 12)

Hours	Species
6.5	water opossum
6.0	giant armadillo
5.5	
5.0	North American opossum
4.5	
4.0	European hedgehog
3.6	cat, big brown bat
3.0	ground squirrel, nine banded armadillo, golden hamster
2.5	rat, mountain beaver, desert hedgehog, East American mole, tree shrew
2.0	African giant pouched rat, star nosed mole, little brown bat, mole-rat, tenrec, red fox
1.5	man, pig, owl monkey, chinchilla, Asian elephant, grey seal, phalanger
1.0	mouse, galago, rhesus monkey, okapi, chimpanzee, Brazilian tapir
0.5	cow, goat, guinea pig, vervet, tree (and rock) hyrax, horse, patas monkey, rabbit, sheep, baboon
less than 0.5	giraffe

are well hidden. Others such as man, cats and chimpanzees are relatively secure because they are strong and aggressive. Man, as we have already seen, also takes great care not to sleep in exposed places. It can also be argued that animals at the bottom of the league table are relatively insecure when asleep. This is obviously true of timid and exposed grazing animals such as sheep and cows. It may also be true of the guinea baboon which sleeps very precariously as far out along the branches of the tree as it dares go. This sleep site reduces the danger from predators but increases the danger of falling to the ground.

Of course we could argue for a long time about which animals are secure, and which insecure, while asleep but Allison and Van Twyver have offered more evidence. They compared the sleep of five rodent species, hamsters, squirrels, rats, chinchillas and mice.[5] These animals show similar amounts of sleep (between 12.5 hours and 14.5 hours) but they have dramatic differences in the amount of AS they enjoy. They found that large amounts of AS were associated with less frequent awakenings from sleep which suggests that secure sleepers, who wake less often, have more AS and insecure sleepers, who wake frequently, have relatively little AS.

These findings agree very nicely with the observation that AS episodes very often finish with a brief awakening. This has been specifically reported for the rat, hedgehog and rabbit, animals which show intermediate amounts of AS. Man and the cat, which show a lot of AS, do not usually wake after AS periods. However, Langford, Pearson and I[6] have found that people are more likely to wake from AS than QS and that when they do wake from AS, this frequently terminates the AS episode altogether. Such findings have given rise to the idea that AS is a fragile state which gives way readily to wakefulness, especially if the animal has cause to be afraid.

It is certainly true that temporary anxiety can cause a dramatic reduction in AS. For example, when animals are brought into the laboratory for studying, their sleep is often very broken and the proportion of AS which can be recorded is negligible although QS is seen for long periods. After exposure to the laboratory, as the animal gradually acclimatises, normal sleep returns with regular amounts of both states. The reverse effect can be seen in cows who may show substantial periods of AS in the safety of their stalls but this is severely reduced when the cows are sent out grazing, where, presumably, they feel more exposed. Human volunteers also show a large reduction in AS time on their first night in the sleep laboratory even though total sleep time is only slightly less. This effect, which probably affects us all when sleeping in strange beds, rapidly disappears after a few nights in the same bed.

The basic finding is that AS is reduced under strange or anxiety provoking situations but is present at normal levels under familiar, safe surroundings. When using rabbits, new to the laboratory, an experimenter may expect to wait days or even months before observing AS. However, Fauré advises the following environmental conditions to speed its appearance; silence, warmth, low illumination, the absence of members of the opposite sex, sufficient food of adequate moistness and the smell of its own near-by excrement![7]

Other researchers have shown that AS is particularly sensitive to a cold or excessively warm environment. If cats are exposed to prolonged severe cold or heat they will still sleep but AS will be reduced or absent for the first few days before returning slowly to normal levels.[8] Bats also show a reduction in AS in response to cold although, unlike the cat, they do not fight the cold by maintaining a high body temperature throughout.

Most drugs which affect the central nervous system similarly cause a reduction in the proportion of AS. Barbiturates and alcohol, for example, cause an increase in total sleep time but a reduction in AS time. This effect gradually disappears over a number of nights, if the drugs are taken regularly. Some drugs have a less severe effect than others and modern sleeping pills are often chosen as much for their ability to provide a normal pattern of sleep states as for their ability to induce sleep in the first place.

It may be that drugs exert special effects on the sleep-control mechanisms or it may be that drugs are just another stress on the system like anxiety or severe heat and cold. It certainly seems, however, that AS is very sensitive to such stresses and that it responds to them by either disappearing or by occurring in much shorter episodes, at least at the beginning of the stressful period. These findings confirm the notion that AS is a *fragile* state. Only continued research will tell us just how fragile it is, or under what circumstances this fragility is most marked.

The depth of sleep

It is reasonable to ask at this point, 'which is the deeper type of sleep?' While the question sounds simple enough, I have never heard a simple answer. For one thing it depends on how you measure depth. Langford, Pearson and I found that human volunteers were more likely to wake spontaneously from AS than from QS. So in one sense, at least, AS is a lighter stage of sleep. When we tried waking them using buzzers and tape recordings of someone calling their name, we found little difference between AS and light QS.[9] We did, however, find that volunteers were very slow to wake from deep QS which occurs during the first few hours of sleep. Our findings agree well with the results from other laboratories.

Students of animal sleep find a very different pattern. Using non-human mammals and birds, almost all experiments show that it is much more difficult to rouse a creature from AS than from QS. This result is opposite to the human data. There is, of course, no complication here, arising from differences between light and deep QS, because QS is present only in the 'deep' variety among most animal species. It is something of a mystery why human and animal sleepers should be different. It is clear, however, that non-human animals show the majority pattern while human experiments are revealing a somewhat abnormal pattern. One possible explanation is that human volunteers are usually expected to perform a learned action, such as pressing a button, while animals are simply allowed to perform a natural reaction, such as opening the eyes or even just stirring. It could be that learned reactions require a much clearer state of mind and that this is more likely to follow an arousal from AS. Some support for this view comes from one of the few experiments using rats which required that the animal perform a learned response. Van Twyver and Garrett[10] woke rats up with a signal which normally warned of an impending electric shock. This shock could only be avoided by running to another part of the box which they were housed in. They found that the rats were less likely to wake up out of AS (as expected) but that, if they did wake from AS, they were much more likely to run away to avoid the shock than if they had woken from QS!

The general finding, therefore, is that AS is much less easily disturbed in animals and birds. Human data do not follow the same pattern but this may be explained in terms of the different measuring techniques. On the other hand, it may also be true that we are just plain different. Only future research will tell.

Sleep before birth

Another reason for avoiding the term 'dreaming sleep' comes from studies of the sleep of newborn babies and of animals which are still in the womb. This research shows that AS is very plentiful both soon after and soon before birth. It is so plentiful that some experts have even suggested that the main purpose of AS is to promote the healthy development of the brain in the helpless infant by providing a substitute, during sleep, for the stimulation which the babies would have, when awake, if they were not restricted in the womb. While there is no direct evidence in favour of this theory, it does offer an explanation for some of these facts which any other theory will also have to deal with.

There are many problems in attempting to trace the development of sleeping patterns in infants because of the differences in brain electrical activity between babies and adults. Nevertheless, careful and scholarly analysis of the records of newborn babies, both full term and premature, have helped build up a general picture of this development which is confirmed by studies of animals such as lambs and calves, both before and after birth.

Before the brain has matured fully, there may be no electrical indication of waking or sleeping patterns. When these do emerge, however, the earliest kind of sleep to appear has more in common with AS than QS. This has given rise to the general belief that AS appears first in developing animals. As the patterns become easier to interpret, it is soon obvious that AS occupies a very large proportion of infant sleep which itself occupies a large proportion of the day. For example, a new-born baby sleeps for roughly sixteen hours each day and roughly half of this is made up of AS, compared with only one-fifth which is the adult proportion. The sleep of premature babies has an even higher percentage of AS. A newborn kitten may sleep for even longer and it can spend up to 90 per cent of its sleep in AS which is much more than the 24 per cent reported for the adult cat.

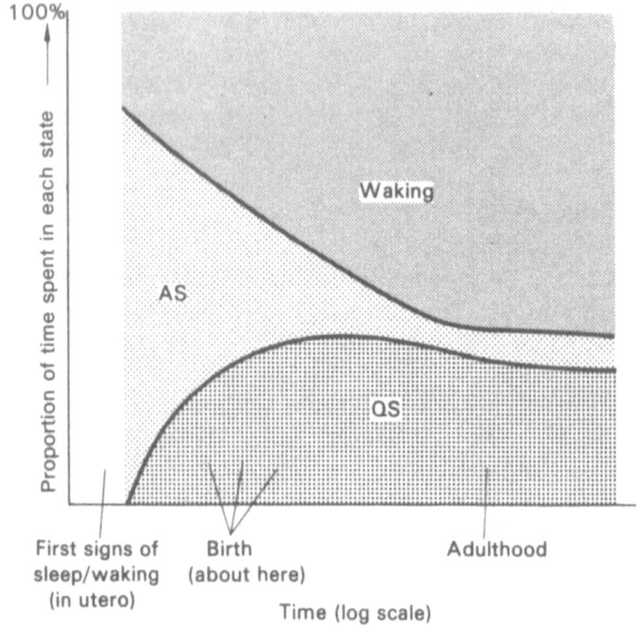

Figure 5.3 The ontogeny of sleep
This general scheme illustrates changes in the proportions of active and quiet sleep among mammals as a function of age. A log scale is used for age because only minor changes occur after infancy.

As the animal matures, it usually comes to sleep less and less. This drop in sleeping-time is made up mainly of a reduction in AS because the amounts of QS fall off only slightly after rising to a later peak in infancy. Figure 5.3 offers a schematic version of the pattern which seems to apply to the animal species which have been studied so far.

Once again we are faced with exciting new evidence which makes us think of AS as a special state of the organism. Its existence seems to offer implications far beyond the nature and significance of dreaming. So far, no very good explanation of the need, if any, for this special state has yet emerged. In the next chapter I shall offer my own, heretical views which attempt to deal with all of these strange observations. In particular, I hope to show that there is reason to reject all notions of any special physical or mental need for dreaming sleep. Moreover, I will suggest that, in principle at least, AS is just as much an evolutionary hangover as QS, playing no vital role in the life of modern civilised man.

6 The origin of dreaming sleep

There are three main types of theory of active sleep which currently dominate the international research scene.[1] The first type suggests that AS exists in order to exercise the brain at intervals during sleep. The discovery of massive amounts of AS in babies both before and after birth inspired one version of this theory which points to the many possible advantages of exercising the immature brain before it meets the challenge of reality. Another version suggests that long periods of quiet sleep may be harmful to the brain even in adults and that AS may have arrived to counteract these effects by producing at regular intervals short periods of excited pseudo-wakefulness.

The second type of theory suggests that AS permits some special type of recovery which cannot take place as effectively during wakefulness or QS. There are an enormous number of such theories suggesting different kinds of recovery from the mental to the biochemical. Each theory is supported by one or two experiments, usually from the theorists' own laboratory, but few theories have found support from a wide range of experiments as we might reasonably require. The general idea that *some* kind of recovery is taking place during AS was mainly inspired by the 'dream deprivation' studies whose findings of irritability and increased aggression following lack of AS have not been reproduced in recent experiments (see chapter 4).

The third type of theory emphasises the biological advantages of the brief awakening which occurs at the end of an AS episode in many species. Snyder, a prominent American contributor to the scientific literature on sleep, has said that these awakenings give the animal a chance to survey its surroundings for predators. In this respect AS is considered to serve a vigilance function.

Unfortunately there is very little experimental evidence which directly supports the theory, but it is an intriguing hypothesis none the less.

These three types of theory have two major drawbacks. First they each explain only some of the facts and, second, none of the three are supported by evidence which proves, beyond reasonable doubt, that AS is, or ever was, really essential for the survival of mammals and birds generally. We know that sleep is controlled by a complex mechanism which regulates the average amount of sleep we have and which carefully switches in and out the two major types of sleep according to a regular, pre-programmed sequence. We assume that the complex structure of sleep must have arisen in the course of evolution to solve some crucial survival problem. In other words, all of the bird and mammal species who did not have this fancy sleep pattern must have perished, leaving only those who did. The real question facing us now is, 'why did they die?'. I am not convinced that any of the three above theories offers us a convincing answer to this question.

The perspective of evolution

It is generally believed that AS is a newcomer on the sleep scene, and that QS, or some version of it, has been with us since time immemorial. Questions concerning the evolution of AS are usually based on this assumption. Thus, we might want to know what was so wrong with QS that it needed to be supplemented by AS. All three of the types of theory described above are usually presented in terms of an answer to this question.

In fact, there is no very good reason to assume that AS is any more recent an innovation than QS. It is true that observations of reptiles and fish have not yielded any reports of regularly occurring episodes of rapid-eye-movements, but neither have they produced any convincing evidence of what we know of as QS. Reptilian sleep, or quiescence, is a fairly simple affair, according to the reports, with very little by way of change from beginning to end. We can be certain that it is not the two-state affair which we see so clearly in birds and mammals. We feel confident that our sleep most likely evolved from something very similar to the

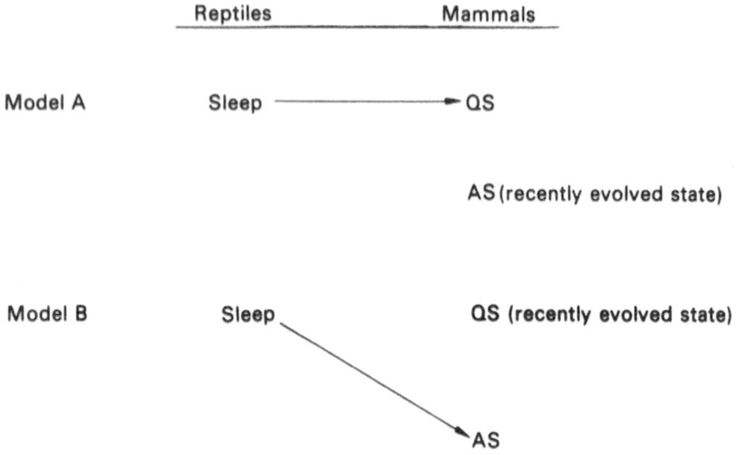

Figure 6.1 Two alternative models of the evolution of mammalian sleep states.

one-state sleep of modern reptiles but we cannot be certain whether the reptilian sleep state gave rise directly to our AS or QS.

Figure 6.1 illustrates the two possibilities I have in mind. Model A describes the popular belief that our QS is a modified version of reptilian sleep, while AS is new. Model B describes the heretical view that our AS is a modified version of reptilian sleep, while QS is new. I shall be arguing in favour of this heresy for the rest of the chapter because it will lead us to a very simple and compelling explanation of the evolution of QS and the complex alternating structure of the sleep patterns of birds and mammals. Of course, it is always possible that AS and QS are both new states and have nothing to do with reptilian quiescence which we left behind many millions of years ago. This is a somewhat uneconomical explanation which I shall disregard until someone gives me a good reason to take it seriously.

Evolution and infant development

My main reason for adopting such an unpopular theory, springs not from comparative animal studies at all but from the observation, mentioned in the last chapter, that AS appears to be the first sleep state to appear in the development of infants. When studying the development of the unborn baby, it is not uncommon to find that many features appear in the order of their original evolution. This is a highly reasonable state of affairs if we pause to consider how the development of the embryo is controlled by the genetic blueprint which it inherits from its parents. It is as if great cathedrals were always built by slowly modifying a small church making it gradually bigger and more magnificent with annexes, decorations and gradual structural alterations. This method might be chosen because the first cathedral was built in this way and the stonemasons knew that their plan worked. So it is with the human body, which is built to a plan which has arisen over millions of years of gradual modification of simpler life forms. By careful observation of the stages of development, while still in the womb, we can often gain insight into the gradual evolution, over millions of years, of the detailed architectural plan.

The prior arrival of AS during infant development does not prove that AS evolved before QS but it does make it very plausible. Certainly I have found very little reason to reject the idea that AS evolved first. It is true that reptilian sleep does not show sustained rapid-eye-movements but neither does the sleep of all mammals or birds. Reptiles do, however, show brain electrical rhythms which are broadly similar to wakefulness and this is certainly a reliable feature of AS in mammals and birds. Muscle tension which is sometimes, but not always, low during AS in mammals and birds is also very low during reptilian sleep. On the other hand, there are no major similarities between QS and reptilian sleep. Beyond this point the argument becomes technical and confused and I do not intend to pursue the details here. Let it suffice to say that, as matters stand, we can make a reasonable case that the existing evidence is not grossly inconsistent with the idea that AS in mammalian sleep evolved directly from reptilian sleep.

The origin of QS

If AS has the longer evolutionary history, as I am proposing, we shall now need to ask why QS evolved to supplement it. What vital ingredient was missing from AS that was supplied by the new

QS? Why is it that reptiles can survive without QS, when birds and mammals apparently cannot? We might also be interested to know why AS and QS should need to alternate throughout the sleep period. Why not have one long period of AS followed by one long period of QS?

The answers may lie in the results of a series of experiments reported by Parmeggiani and Rabini,[2] two Italian researchers working at the University of Bologna in Italy. They observed the sleep of cats when they were exposed for short periods to various environmental temperatures. They found that time spent in QS was not markedly affected by extremes of heat or cold whereas time spent in AS was substantially reduced. At temperatures below freezing or at approximately body heat, AS all but disappeared. It was as if the cats could not cope with the stress during AS. If the very low temperatures were maintained over a number of days then the proportion of AS was observed to remain at a much reduced level throughout.

Parmeggiani and Rabini also noticed that the cat's normal responses to heat or cold stress did not operate normally during AS. During QS shivering was observed in response to cold and panting in response to heat but neither of these responses were observed during AS. It is very important to all warm-blooded animals such as birds and mammals that they maintain a normal body temperature at all times. Shivering and panting are two of the various methods which are available to an animal to raise or lower its temperature, to compensate for changes in its environment. If, for some reason, these vital processes do not work properly during AS, it is clear that the animal must respond by suppressing AS as much as possible, or run the risk of a lethal dose of hypothermia or hyperthermia.

This could be the answer we need to explain why animals with an AS/QS cycle have survived and those without it have perished. Reptiles do not attempt to regulate their body temperature while they are asleep. They simply allow it to float up and down according to the dictates of the environment. Mammals and birds must do so and they developed special techniques for doing so during wakefulness. It is possible, however, that we inherited a sleep pattern from our reptilian ancestors which was not flexible enough to permit such regulation. This meant that long periods of sleep would be highly undesirable and even dangerous under conditions of extreme heat or cold. Short periods would not have proved too troublesome because the body takes some time to cool down (or heat up), especially if a protected sleep site has been carefully chosen. Nevertheless, sleep length would need to be measured in terms of minutes rather than hours and regular periods of wakefulness would be required to permit the animal to restore normal body temperatures.

If this analysis is correct, we might expect that the earliest warm-blooded mammals might have developed a sleep pattern which consisted of short periods of sleep (AS) which alternated with longer periods of wakefulness. This pattern would have had the advantage that the animal was able to take meals all round the clock. This may even have been essential in the earliest warm-blooded species because of the enormous expenditure of energy associated with maintaining a high body temperature. Nevertheless, such a sleep pattern would mean that the animals would lose all of the advantages to be gained by long periods of immobility discussed at length earlier (chapter 2).

It is possible that QS evolved specifically to preserve the continuity of sleep by filling the gaps between periods of active sleep in a way which preserved immobility while at the same time permitting temperature regulation. This, in itself, would explain why the two-state pattern of sleep is restricted to warm-blooded animals. It would also explain why periods of QS are interspersed between short periods of AS. Clearly, there would be little point in having all of QS concentrated in a single episode, since its main function is to fill the gaps between periods of AS which would otherwise be filled by wakefulness.

This new theory offers a single, very good reason why QS should have evolved to supplement AS in a new two-state sleep pattern. Warm-blooded animals were able to survive and even thrive because of the many advantages conferred upon them by the ability to remain active and effective in a wide range of environmental temperatures. They were able to do this only because of the development of a number of special temperature-regulating abilities which included panting, shivering, sweating, changing the arrangement of body hairs and controlling the flow of blood near the surface of the skin. It was important that these systems should function as effectively during sleep as waking. In fact they did not function well during the sleep state inherited from reptiles, which accordingly could only be sustained for a matter of minutes. To maintain immobility between such brief episodes a new kind of sleep (QS) was introduced which did permit thermoregulation.

A new perspective

Since Parmeggiani's work, further confirmation of the failure of thermoregulatory mechanisms during AS in mammals has come from California where a team of researchers - Heller, Glotzbach, Berger and Walker,[3] using very sophisticated techniques - have shown that the ground squirrel does not respond to cold stress during AS by increasing its energy expenditure, even though it does so normally during QS and wakefulness. We clearly need to know more about this phenomenon before we can attempt any precise analysis of the full reasons justifying the evolution of QS. Nevertheless, we already have a new approach which may prove more valuable than existing theories when trying to make sense of the available evidence.

For the first time, I find that I have a convincing explanation for the strange relationship between the weight of an animal and the length of the AS/QS cycle. In figure 5.2 we saw that the interval between the onset of successive episodes of AS was long for heavy animals but short for small animals. This means that small animals such as the hamster may have more AS than large animals like the chimpanzee, but the hamster must take it in the form of many small episodes while the chimp has relatively few but long periods. A chimpanzee has only 7 AS episodes per day, each of roughly 21 minutes duration (total 147 minutes), while a hamster has about 50 AS episodes per day, each approximately 4 minutes long (total 202 minutes). This can readily be understood in terms of the dangers of the failure of thermoregulation during AS. The chimpanzee is a large, bulky animal whose body temperature would fall, or rise, only slowly in the absence of any deliberate attempt to regulate it. The hamster, however, is small with a relatively large surface area. For him, cooling can take place very rapidly indeed in a cold atmosphere, if no attempts are made to conserve existing body heat and generate even more. As a result, AS periods can be tolerated only for short periods in small animals.

This leads us to the interesting speculation that the AS/QS cycle evolved initially in heavy warm-blooded animals and was only subsequently to be found in lightweight warm-blooded animals. The reason for this is as follows. It is easy to understand why the cycle should be shortened as animals become lighter because of the increased dangers consequent upon the failure to thermoregulate in smaller creatures. It is not so easy to understand why the cycle should be lengthened for larger animals, since a short AS/QS would not appear to be harmful to them. It makes sense therefore to suggest that the AS/QS cycle first evolved in heavy animals. Fortunately, it became linked to the weight of the animal possibly via the mechanisms which control metabolic rate - which meant that the system could be adapted readily to the smaller descendants of our pioneer two-state sleepers.

It is tempting to believe that all warm-blooded animals are either birds or mammals and this confuses the argument because early mammals are believed to have been very small (like shrews), although the earliest birds may have been quite large. It is important to remember, however, that the techniques of temperature regulation using purely physiological methods must have been perfected by early reptiles who are now extinct. During the early stages of experimentation, the mechanisms were probably most inefficient and unreliable, a state of affairs which would only be tolerable in larger animals whose body temperature changed only slowly under heat or cold stress. This line of argument leads me to suggest that the AS/QS cycle may have been present in large thermoregulating reptiles whose descendants we are.

This suggestion is likely to meet considerable opposition because of the discovery by Allison, Van Twyver and Goff,[4] that the spiny anteater - a primitive egg-laying mammal - does not show AS, even though it is likely that it shares a common reptilian ancestry with other mammals such as ourselves. If the early thermoregulating reptiles bequeathed a two-state sleep pattern to its descendants, why do we show AS and the spiny anteaters show none? It may be, of course, that Allison and his colleagues are wrong in their interpretation of the data. Certainly the sleep patterns which they report do show a regular switching between two states during the animal's immobility period. While one of these states is indubitably QS, they argue that the other state is more like quiet wakefulness than AS, even though the animal does not move at this time. This may boil down to a matter of opinion because AS and quiet wakefulness are very similar anyhow. Alternatively, it may be that sleep in the spiny anteater represents a specialised adaptation to the dangers of heat loss during AS, by retaining the old AS/QS cycle but transforming the AS episodes into something resembling immobile wakefulness in an attempt to thermoregulate all day without interruption. It is significant that spiny anteaters are reported to shiver during quiet wakefulness but not during QS. This may mean that they have adapted to meet some special problem which other mammals do not have to face.

Babies and adults

Our new perspective also allows us to revisit the data on sleep in babies before and after birth. The prior emergence of AS in the foetus is, of course, explained by the fact that AS appeared first in the course of evolution. The early dominance of AS over QS, soon before and soon after birth, may also reflect an early stage in the evolution of the AS/QS two-state sleep pattern but it may also reflect a lack of the need to thermoregulate. In the womb and soon after birth, basking in the warmth of maternal affection, temperature regulation is not a pressing problem and long periods of AS can be tolerated. Very soon, however, the problem will become very pressing and the length of each AS episode - but not the number of episodes - is dramatically reduced during the early weeks of life.

Berger,[5] whose work on thermoregulation in the ground squirrel has already been mentioned, has drawn attention to the parallel development of QS and the ability of an animal to regulate its own body temperature as it grows older. Young animals spend a great deal of their time asleep and it follows that their ability to maintain a steady thermal equilibrium will depend very much upon the proportion of time spent in QS since thermoregulation is defective in AS.

The gradual decrease in the AS proportion of total sleep continues into adulthood, where it is almost always less than 25 per cent, although it can sometimes be considerably less. It is likely that 25 per cent had been found to be the tolerable maximum for any mammalian species and for birds this figure is probably much smaller. We might reasonably ask why AS has not dissappeared altogether now that QS has evolved to enforce immobility with less danger. After all, we know that drugs which suppress AS completely usually produce no obvious consequential ill-effects. The reason probably lies in the fact that animals are well able to handle small amounts of AS which can in any case be even further reduced in emergencies. We would only expect AS to have disappeared, in the course of evolution, if its continued presence militated against the survival of species, which it obviously does not. Moreover, if QS evolved after AS, we can assume that the neural mechanisms which control its switching on and off, would be closely intertwined with the AS control mechanisms. It might be that QS control cannot be sufficiently disentangled from AS control to permit the simple reintroduction of a one-state sleep pattern. The only feasible procedure would be to increase the sleep proportion of QS to as near 100 per cent as possible while retaining vestigial quantities of AS. This is, of course, what has happened to the adult sleep of many species.

Fragility of active sleep

Temperature control problems go only part of the way to explaining the rapid suppression of AS in the face of stress. We can see why time spent in AS should be reduced under conditions of heat or cold stress but why should it also be reduced at times of high anxiety, as we found in chapter 5? Why is it that many animals often finish a period of AS with a brief awakening while this rarely, if ever, happens during the switch from QS to AS?

The answers to these questions are still far from clear, although some clues are available. We saw (p. 82) that AS was generally a deeper sleep state than QS, in the sense that animals are less likely to respond to stimuli which occur during AS. This might be construed either as an advantage or a disadvantage. On the one hand, the purpose of sleep is to preserve immobility which it may do by rendering an animal less reactive to its environment. In that sense, the deeper the sleep, the better it is. On the other hand, there are occasions where a response is imperative, for example, when a predator is about to pick up an animal and carry it off, or when the sleep site is threatened by fire, water or collapse of one kind or another. Too deep a sleep is clearly a disadvantage on such occasions.

Some kind of middle path needs to be steered between the disadvantages of too deep and too light a sleep state. It is possible that AS, in the form inherited from our reptilian ancestors, was too deep. This might prove a problem only when normal security precautions were inadequate, for example, immediately following a number of frightening incidents which indicate that danger is at hand. In such circumstances, it could prove advantageous to suppress AS selectively and rely mainly upon QS for an acceptable level of vigilance during the immobility period. Of course, if the threat is very severe, the only procedure is to suppress sleep altogether, which is what usually occurs. This approach would certainly agree with Allison and Van Twyver's observation (p. 79) that animals who were typically more exposed to danger during sleep, slept less and enjoyed a smaller proportion of AS than other animals.

The tendency of certain animals, such as rats, rabbits and rhesus monkeys, to terminate AS periods with brief arousals is not well developed in all animals. It is certainly much less obvious in man and cats. Nevertheless, it occurs often enough to require an explanation. Once again this will not prove too easy but the new perspective, which requires that AS evolved first, gives us a starting point. We must imagine a transition period, far back in evolutionary history, when AS was coming to be a nuisance but before QS had been invented. The only way to minimise the dangers of the heat loss, or loss of vigilance which occurred during sleep was to arrange to wake up at regular intervals. As a result, the earliest versions of the sleep-control machinery were designed to terminate sleep after a fixed period. If this feature of the machine is still operating today, we might expect a brief arousal to follow all AS periods, even though QS moves in quickly to take over control until the time is ripe for another episode of AS.

The question needs now to be changed to ask why these arousals are not obvious in all mammals. The answer to this new question may simply be that these arousals are suppressed in secure mammals who no longer have much to gain from the additional vigilance which recurrent arousals offer. It is to Snyder we owe this idea that these brief arousals allow an anxious animal to scan its environment regularly for signs of danger during sleep. Although this seems to be obviously advantageous, there is still a lack of experimental evidence to support the idea that animals actually do make use of these arousals in this way. Until this is forthcoming we need to be cautious.

Another possibility is that animals need to wake up to find out if they are hungry, cold, wet, have a full bladder, etc. Regular arousals would certainly be helpful and, if there were no problems requiring attention, sleep could return promptly and the immobility period continue as if nothing had happened. Small mammals would benefit more from this device because they need to eat more frequently than large mammals, and the consequences of prolonged dampness or cold are more dramatically serious for them. Human adults are not likely to starve from oversleeping but the problem is serious for the human newborn, who should be fed roughly once every three hours. Since babies sleep for up to twenty hours per day, missing a few vital feeds in a row might be a real danger. The human infant has an AS episode once every hour and it could be that the arousals which follow each episode are used to assess hunger level. If this is the case, and it remains to be established firmly, then we have an explanation for the infant three-hour feeding rhythm, as Kleitman has suggested, since each feeding cycle consists of three or four QS/AS cycles strung together with a short arousal after each AS period and a long arousal after the third, or fourth, when the baby is hungry and demands to be fed.

Body functions during AS

When AS was first discovered, a great deal of attention was devoted to the changes in various physiological functions which could be easily measured. These included a waking type of brain electrical activity, a drop in the tension of the main postural muscles, irregular fluctuations of systolic blood pressure and heart and respiration rates, twitching of the extremities (paws or hands), rapid-eye-movements, increased peristalsis of the stomach and penile erections. It was hoped that these observations would prove clues to the real nature and purpose of dreaming sleep, but this did not happen. If anything, the problem simply became more difficult to solve as additional facts accumulated.

It is not clear whether the new theory of the origins of AS will help us to explain this odd collection of physiological facts. Some speculations are probably not out of order, however. First, the low levels of muscle tension during AS may simply be a direct hand-down from reptilian sleep which is characterised by a complete absence of muscle tension. In fact, the suppression of muscle activity may be an important element in the reptilian mechanisms for suppressing action during periods of quiescence. This is unfortunate for mammals because the heat generated from muscle tension is valuable for maintaining a high body temperature. This is especially true of the large postural muscles. It is therefore possible that the twitching of extremities (including rapid-eye-movements) may constitute relatively feeble attempts to compensate for the lack of heat generated by the postural muscles. It is difficult to attach too much weight to this explanation in view of the very small amount of heat generated by small muscle twitches but it should be considered as a possibility.

Irregularities of cardiovascular control functions are also difficult to explain. It may be that this also reflects a pattern descended from reptilian sleep. During QS, heart and respiration are certainly much more regular and, if we accept the idea that QS is a relatively new state, this might be seen as an improvement. Heart rate and blood flow data during sleep in reptiles are not readily obtainable and such as are available do not necessarily indicate anything like the irregularity found during mammalian AS. Nevertheless, it is worth considering the possibility that the fluctuations of respiration and heart rate represent a reduction in the nicety of control which is normally exercised by higher centres during wakefulness. This may also apply to penile erections and changes in stomach activity which take place during AS. Instead of looking for some purpose to explain the erratic nature of these functions, we might be better advised to treat the phenomenon in terms of a failure of control by higher centres, a failure which has been compensated by the introduction of the new and preferred state of QS.

Studies of domestic animals such as cows and sheep offer further evidence in favour of the general theory that AS has been suppressed by mammals because it is inappropriate to their life style. Many years of outstanding research by French physiologists into the sleep and waking patterns of farm animals have revealed that the rumination, a vital digestive function, continues from wakefulness into drowsiness and then into QS only to stop abruptly at the onset of AS. They have also discovered that the nasolabial secretions which keep the lips and nose of the cow continuously moist, stop suddenly at the onset of AS causing a rapid drying of this area and a dramatic rise in the local skin temperature. It is not surprising that the cow and the sheep have exceptionally short AS periods (considering their size) and that AS occupies a relatively small proportion of their total immobility period.

The evidence of body function changes during AS points toward a breakdown of a number of physiological functions of special survival value to mammals. The data for birds are too scanty as yet to permit any conclusions. There is evidence that animals fail to thermoregulate during AS and that ruminants fail to ruminate. Many experiments have shown that arousal thresholds are especially high during AS, resulting in a loss of vigilance, and the erratic performance of simple functions such as blood flow and respiration suggest that their careful control, witnessed during QS, had been abandoned. It is as if early mammals developed the ability to regulate these functions during waking but not sleep and that they developed a new kind of sleep (QS) to replace the old and defective AS. This replacement process was not completed, however, and we witness today in almost all mammals a regular alternation of the two states. Among adult mammals the proportion of sleep occupied by AS is usually less than 25 per cent and in times of stress - whether caused by anxiety or physical discomfort - this value may be substantially reduced even, exceptionally, to the point where it is briefly absent altogether.

The evolutionary sequence

An attempt had been made to sketch a rough plan of the evolution of the AS/QS sleep pattern from its simple reptilian origins. This

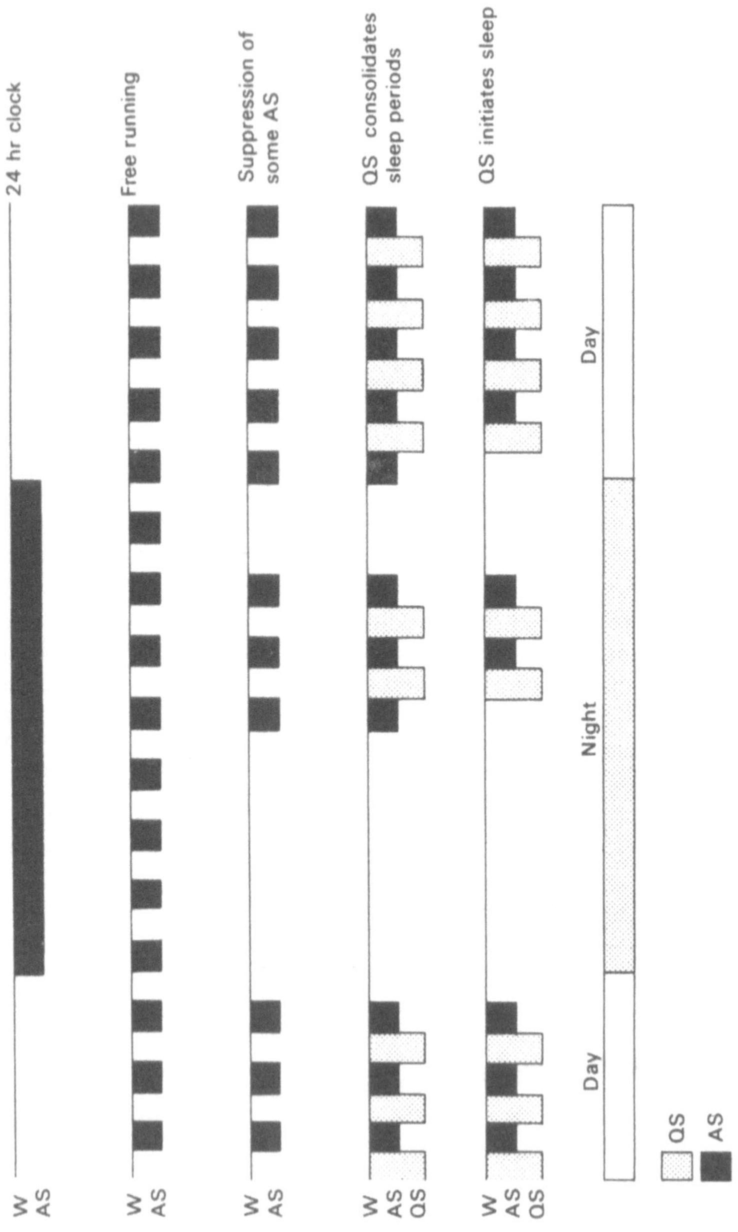

Figure 6.2 Evolution of the QS/AS Sleep Cycle

is shown in Figure 6.2. The top line of the diagram represents the sleep of a primitive reptile who slept at night and was active by day. The second line shows a possible scheme for the sleep of one of its earliest warm-blooded descendants. The sleep period is broken up into short periods - because of the failure of thermoregulation mechanisms during sleep. It may be that this regular pattern was driven by some kind of internal metabolic clock which is a speeded up version of the twenty-four-hour clock which controlled the sleep-waking patterns of its ancestor. Line three shows a suppression of some sleep periods which allowed the animal to concentrate its foraging for food in the relatively safe night time. QS is introduced in line four to consolidate adjacent periods of AS into long periods of immobility By this time it is assumed that the animal can tolerate long periods between meals and can therefore remain hidden for most of the daylight hours.

In line five, a small change is made, to cause the sleep period always to begin with a period of QS rather than AS. It is not clear why it should happen, but it is true to say that all adult mammals so far studied, with the exception of the seal, begin their sleep with a substantial period of QS. It may be that QS is more effective than AS in producing a rapid conversion from sleep to wakefulness. It is certainly true that reptiles fall asleep only very gradually, even after prolonged sleep deprivation, while mammals can fall asleep in a matter of minutes.

It may seem rather odd to suggest that the evolutionary sequence went through a stage where sleep normally began with an AS period. It is, of course, essential to the theory that QS evolved to fill the gaps between adjacent AS periods, and it is supported by studies of infant sleep which shows that, for the first three months of life, sleep normally begins with AS.[6] Later in the first year of life, the normal adult sequence becomes dominant. So far this detail has received very little attention because it cannot be explained by any existing theory. However, if we accept the idea that the sequence of development observed in babies reflects the sequence of changes which occurred in the course of evolution, then we have an interesting piece of evidence which offers preliminary support for the suggested change between lines four and five in Figure 6.2.

The evolutionary sequence required by my theory of the nature and function of AS in mammals departs from orthodox theories so radically that we should not expect it to receive too enthusiastic a reception. Indeed, it calls into question so very many cherished notions concerning dreaming sleep, that a healthy scepticism is really the only appropriate response. It is certainly true that many of the details of the theory must be wrong because they are only guesses based upon incomplete evidence which, in any case, was collected to be used as answers to different questions. Nevertheless, I have been pleasantly surprised at how many different, and hitherto perplexing, phenomena have yielded to explanation as a result of extensions of the simple idea that AS evolved before QS and not the other way around.

7 Insomnia

Dear Sir,

I unfortunately am one of the lack of sleep people. I never go to sleep before two or three a.m. and some nights I don't sleep at all, but I find that I am feeling very sick next day and unwell. My doctor told me this was caused by the body not having any rest all night. I have had difficulty sleeping now for fifteen to sixteen years . . . .

Yours,
Mrs G. W.

P.S When I sleep I dream a lot.

Dear Sir,

I am 48 years old. I have never slept a wink for years. Although I have had tablets I have never slept . . . . I toss and turn, curse and blind, talking to myself because I cannot sleep. Oh! how I would love a nights sleep for once . . . . I still find time to be jolly and welcome people into my home but I would give anything for a nights sleep.

Yours truly,
Mrs M. E. H.

Dear Sir,

Ever since childhood I have suffered from bad, disturbed sleep. I wake in the morning in an exhausted state, instead of feeling refreshed. It takes me some hours to recover from this wretched condition and to get back to something approaching normality . . . . I have been to many doctors to become cured of my bad sleep problem, but without success. Among these doctors were several psychiatrists, who gave me psychiatric treatment, all to no avail . . . .

Yours truly,
A. P.

Dear Dr Meddis,

I make every effort to be in bed each night at the latest 10.30 p.m. . . . . The reason for going to bed at this time is that I feel tired and sleepy but directly I get into bed the tiredness seems to go and I cannot get off to sleep for a couple of hours . . . . I enjoy a fairly active life . . . . I am a non smoker, practically a tee-totaller and NEVER take drugs . . . .

I trust you can find some remedy for my sleeplessness as I feel I could really enjoy a really good sound nights sleep.

Yours sincerely,
J. M.

These extracts constitute only a short selection from a very large batch of letters which I received in response to my request for nonsomniacs to come forward. Although the authors of these notes clearly failed to qualify as healthy, happy non-sleepers, I could not help but be impressed by the large number of people who complained of poor sleep and the depth of misery and the intensity of frustration which their letters reflected. I am not medically qualified and therefore there was little I could do beyond offering reassurance and general advice on matters of sleep hygiene. It made me feel very helpless.

In many ways my views on the nature and function of sleep, which were then being publicised in the press, appeared to be making matters worse for these individuals. In particular, my theory that sleep did not serve the purpose of restoration of bodily deficiencies, caused much annoyance among some insomniacs who attributed their ill-health and misery to chronic lack of sleep. To them these ideas were a cruel mockery and their letters were often less than complimentary:

Sir,

You are a Bloody idiot. Have you ever missed any sleep? I wish you suffered from insomnia like I have, going 4–6 nights without sleep. You would then realise what *tripe* you are saying. I bet you have NEVER missed a nights sleep in your life. If you had you would know it makes you that miserable you could bite a nail in half. Somebody should catch hold of you. Tie you up and make you go *A WEEK* WITHOUT sleep. Then see how you feel. You are supposed to be a psychologist. In my opinion you are a Bloody Nut case. A menace to society.

Sleep that off.

In truth, it was not my intention to hurt these people. I do not believe, and have never said, that insomnia is an imaginary ailment. Nor do I deny the agony of the complaint. Although I normally enjoy good sleep, like most people I have suffered from bouts of poor sleep which have made me fully aware of the intensity of suffering which chronic insomniacs experience as a regular feature of their lives. Insomnia is one of the most common ailments presented for treatment to the general practitioner. Moreover it is an ailment least likely to receive satisfactory treatment.

Much of the misunderstanding arises from the belief that there is only one explanation for the suffering of insomniacs. This idea is clear in the first letter quoted above where the doctor is supposed to have attributed the lady's feelings of sickness to a lack of rest during the night. Of course, no one would deny the value of rest as a means of overcoming fatigue but the implication of the doctor's remark is that there is a special quality of rest during sleep which is especially valuable in helping us recover from the ravages of the previous day. According to this view, insomniacs suffer from the lack of this special kind of rest and as a result do not feel fully refreshed in the morning. It follows that the appropriate treatment is to dispense pills which will hopefully increase the amount of sleep which they get.

The immobilisation theory denies that there is anything special about the rest which people enjoy during sleep. It is my own view that sleep-rest may even be inferior in many cases to quiet wakeful relaxation. Mental and physical tensions can be very great in sleep even though we are unaware of it at the time. We do get a glimpse of this turmoil, however, when we experience or witness frightening dreams, night terrors, sleep-walking and tooth grinding. It is only a glimpse because the internal conflicts of sleep only occasionally erupt into wakefulness or visible symptoms. These are the tip of the iceberg.

The immobilisation theory adopts a non-traditional approach. Instead of attributing the agony of insomnia to a lack of normal sleep, it sees the problem in terms of the unpleasantness of an excess of poor quality sleep. The sleep instinct manipulates our wishes so that we come to desire sleep in the late evening. If, for some reason, sleep does not come we experience frustration and a further mounting desire for sleep. During the night when we wake, the sleep instinct continues to operate by specifying a strong desire to go back to sleep. If, for some reason, sleep does not come, we experience more frustration and even feelings of desperation. The sleep mechanism is tuned to enforce a fixed average amount of sleep per twenty-four hours. If our actual average sleep-time is less than that prescribed by the mechanism, we are likely to experience symptoms of mild sleep deprivation. These include reduced motivation, drowsiness, poor concentration and irritability. Such symptoms are probably not troublesome to individuals who enjoy full, exciting lives because the stimulating character of their activities will substantially counteract the reduced motivation. For others, however, these symptoms may result in a definite reduction in their capacity to enjoy life.

We can express the immobilisation view a little more succinctly. Although sleep is of no immediate physiological benefit, no harm results from it, as long as a sleep session runs its normal course. If, however, the sleep mechanism fails to produce sleep at the time when the sleep instinct instils a desire for it, we experience various degrees of frustration. If a malfunction of the mechanism persists for a number of nights we shall suffer the debilitating effects of repeated frustration which become compounded with the symptoms of mild sleep deprivation. The unpleasantness of insomnia may not, therefore, result from a lack of the restorative benefits of sleep but from a disturbance of the smooth functioning of the sleep mechanism, producing unpleasant side effects.

Insomnia, a complicated illness

This explanation is a little too simple to embrace all cases of insomnia and it may be profitable to spend a little time looking at the phenomenon itself. Like most common complaints, insomnia turns out to be a very complex problem with subtle but significant variations from patient to patient. It is tempting to think of insomnia simply as the consequences of lack of sleep but here we are confusing the symptoms with the explanation. The important issue really concerns the reasons why people complain about lack of sleep.

An examination of my post bag reveals two basic and possibly separable problems. On the one hand, there are complaints which are based upon the unpleasantness of not being able to enjoy a 'deep refreshing sleep'. On the other hand, there are complaints which concern the effects of disturbed sleep on mood and performance during the following day. Often people complain of both but quite frequently correspondents complain of only disturbed sleep and specifically say that day-time symptoms are not a problem. The second letter in our selection above illustrates a common theme. The lady is healthy and happy during the day but finds her inability to sleep easily and deeply a profoundly irritating experience.

Complaints about the quality of sleep may take many forms. Some insomniacs believe that they get no sleep at all, some say that they lie awake for hours before falling asleep, others say that they wake often during the night and are unable to go quickly back to sleep and yet others claim to wake very early in the morning and are unable to get much more sleep before the normal time for rising. Some report all of these things while others may simply suffer from only one, such as early waking. It is common also to hear people complain that their sleep is spoiled by dreams. For all of these people their one agreed desire is to have a night of deep, dreamless, and uninterrupted sleep.

It is certainly possible that the different symptoms may indicate a failure of different aspects of the sleep mechanism. For example, the inability of patients to fall asleep at the beginning of the night may reflect a very different malfunction from that responsible for premature early-morning wakings. Similarly, the high incidence of dream recall may reflect either frequent awakenings from dreaming episodes or the intensification of the dreaming process which we know to occur during withdrawal from certain addictive drugs such as alcohol or barbiturates. The careful analysis of the various types of malfunction involved is obviously one of the first tasks of future research into insomnia.

It is much more difficult to say what are the effects of insomnia on the waking life of patients because their complaints in this respect are so much more vague and varied. Some insomniacs claim that their poor sleep has ruined their health altogether. Others report feeling sick or nauseous. Tension and irritability is also a very common complaint. By far the most frequent, and the most vague, impression obtained is that insomnia drains people of their capacity to be spontaneously happy and to enjoy life to the full. Sometimes individuals complain of drowsiness and a tendency to fall asleep during the day. Although this is probably the most obvious consequence of lack of sleep, it is, in my experience, one of the least common complaints of chronic (i.e. long-term) insomniacs, whereas it is the commonest complaint of a good sleeper who has simply had one or two interrupted nights.

A simple interpretation of these reports is not easy to make because it is difficult to decide whether insomnia is the cause of or the result of ill-health and unhappiness. It is clear that tension and worry are most likely to interfere with the quality of sleep. How then can we say that the insomnia causes the tension when it could be the other way round? To the patient, insomnia may be obviously to blame on the grounds that there is no other explanation of the tension. However, we now know that tension and anxiety can appear spontaneously in someone's life for no obvious reason or that worrying may simply be a characteristic of someone's personality. In the same way ill-health may easily be the cause of poor sleep. When ill-health and insomnia are permanent features of life, it must be very difficult for the individual concerned to know which is the cause and which is the symptom. Nevertheless, it is difficult to escape the conclusion that poor sleep does have effects which carry over into the waking day and that these effects include a reduced capacity for the spontaneous enjoyment of life.

The causes of insomnia

The causes of insomnia are not always easy to ascertain. In some cases it is obvious enough. Hay fever, asthma, coughs and colds are clearly likely to interfere with sleep. Similarly, any kind of pain can be expected to delay sleep onset and extend any awakening which does spontaneously occur during the night.

Tension, anxiety, excitement, depression and worries of all kinds are also serious spoilers of a good sleep. In these cases a cure can only be made if the cause is itself tackled first.

Some of the problems appear to be disorders of sleep itself and these include sleep-walking, sleep-talking, night terrors, nightmares, restless leg syndrome and muscular jerks which occur throughout the night. Once again these may be triggered by conflicts or tensions which have occurred during our waking lives but they may also be simply due to a faulty sleep control apparatus whose repair will need to wait until we become a little more knowledgable concerning the biochemistry and physiology of the control centres.

Some dramatic examples of the failure of the sleep mechanisms have recently been studied in California by Bill Dement and his colleagues and subsequently described under the name of *sleep apnea.*[1] These cases involve patients who actually stop breathing while asleep. This may occur because of an obstruction in the upper airway resulting from muscle relaxation or simply because the diaphragm below the lungs stops drawing in air. In either case the result is a drop in oxygen levels and an increase in the carbon dioxide content of the blood. Fortunately this failure to breathe results in an awakening which permits the restoration of normal breathing allowing the patient to fall asleep again until the next apneic episode. Although this illness has only recently been described, it is Dement's view that it may prove to be a common problem.

Regular emergencies of this nature are clearly capable of severely interfering with sleep but the wonder of this illness is that many sufferers appear to be quite unaware of the cause of their insomnia. Often the arousals which are needed to restore normal breathing are only shallow so that the reason for the awakening is not noticed. Moreover, sufferers have often had this problem for the whole of their life and may have had no cause to believe that their experience is in any way abnormal. The problem may only come to light when their struggles for breath are seen by an informed observer. In such cases it would clearly be unwise to treat the insomniac with heavy doses of barbiturates since a failure to wake may result in death.

Indeed, it is believed by many that the mysterious 'crib deaths', where babies die suddenly with no apparent cause, may well be the result of similar failures of normal breathing during sleep. Drs Christian Guilleminault and Nicole Monod[2] working at the Hôpital Port-Royale in Paris did observe two apneic episodes during sleep in a three-week-old girl who was subsequently found dead in her crib on the night after the second episode. A number of laboratories in Europe and the USA are now pursuing this possiblity as a matter of urgency.

Personality problems

A severe difficulty which faces the scientist in search of a full understanding of insomnia arises in connection with reports that poor sleepers tend to have weak and negative personalities. Doctors and researchers often claim that insomniacs are complainers and hypochondriacs. In the surgery, poor sleepers often appear not to be genuinely ill to the doctor who prescribes sometimes merely to avoid a long interview which would interfere with his schedule. Sleep researchers frequently report that insomniacs are more troublesome and complaining in the laboratory than the normal sleepers who come along for comparison purposes. Some investigations using personality tests have even shown groups of insomniacs to have significantly more dependent and more hypochondriacal personalities than groups of 'normals'. These reports create an atmosphere in which it is easy to dismiss insomnia as a complaint of the imagination; a response which is, of course, less than helpful.

When considering this problem, we must remember that many people suffer from insomnia without complaining. For obvious reasons these people do not often turn up in the doctor's surgery or the sleep research laboratory. As a result, those insomniacs who do come to be studied are more likely to be complainers whereas the comparison group of normal people will not contain such a high number of moaners. This creates a source of bias which makes the reports difficult to interpret. We must treat with great caution the argument that all insomnaics are hypochondriacs.

Nevertheless, we are left with the fact that some insomniacs, perhaps especially those who appear regularly in the doctor's surgery, are given to an excessive degree of self-pity and dependence upon the emotional support of others. Among these there are possibly some who are exaggerating a minor disturbance and some who are merely confused as to how much sleep they are really getting or really need. Nevertheless, I suspect that most of them are genuinely experiencing poor sleep on a regular basis and that this frustration is compounded with their natural tendency to experience depression, misery, exasperation and self-pity. It was noted earlier that the effects of poor sleep can be shrugged off by people who enjoy exciting or fulfilling lives. However, the further reduction in spontaneity and enthusiasm which insomnia induces in people whose lives are already monotonous and lacking in colour, may well be the last straw which breaks the camel's back. Indeed, the response which such individuals make to lack of sleep may appear, at first sight, disproportionate, but it is a cruel error to conclude that their suffering is imaginary.

Difficulties in estimating sleep length

The personality complication is seriously compounded by the discovery that sleepers, normal and insomniac, are very poor at estimating how long it takes to fall asleep intially and how much time is spent awake during the night. Thus a 10–30 minute delay to sleep onset can easily be remembered next morning as 30 minutes or 2 minutes. Similarly, 15 minutes of wakefulness during the night may either be forgotten entirely or be assessed as anywhere up to 3 hours. At the time of writing we are, as it happens, analysing the responses of one healthy girl, who falls asleep almost as soon as her head touches the pillow. On one night she was slow to fall asleep, taking a full 4 minutes in all, and next morning she estimated that it took her 45 minutes! Usually she fell asleep sooner than this but her average estimate over eight nights was still approximately 15 minutes. During the night she experienced an average of 13 minutes of wakefulness but her average estimate was approximately 40 minutes.

The cause of this tendency to exaggerate is not difficult to find. After all we have no memories of being asleep, only memories of being awake. Any estimate of how good our sleep was must therefore depend largely upon our memories of waking, not sleeping. This is made even more difficult by the fact that there is no obvious dividing line between sleep and waking. We continue thinking our thoughts after falling asleep although in a more vague and loosely organised fashion. It is quite common for people who have been sleeping soundly for 30 minutes to claim, when woken, that they were not asleep at all but merely lying thinking.

There is a great deal of room for error in our estimates of how much time we spend asleep each night. Recent evidence indicates that this margin for error leads to a consistent exaggeration of sleep loss by regular insomniacs while normal sleepers may either make under- or over-estimates. Frankel[3] an American investigator, studied the sleep of eighteen chronic insomniacs who each came to the laboratory for five successive nights. Another group of eighteen normal sleepers, matched for age and sex with the insomniacs, were simultaneously studied for comparison purposes. On each morning everyone was asked to estimate how long they lay before falling asleep and how much time they had spent sleeping. The results were very revealing.

Normal sleepers estimated their time to fall asleep with high average accuracy while the chronic insomniacs exaggerated the delay by 27 minutes. Similarly, the insomniac group *under-estimated* their real sleep time by a whole half-hour. The normals, on the other hand, also made an average half-hour error in their estimates of total sleep time but this time *on the optimistic side* - they exaggerated the amount of sleep they had had! In fact the insomniac group averaged 40 minutes less sleep than normals by objective criteria. This means that if the insomniacs and normals had swapped impressions in the morning, it would have *seemed* as if the poor sleeper had enjoyed 1 hour 40 minutes less sleep than the normal sleeper even though the time difference was only 40 minutes. It is clear that the problems of estimating sleeping-time may have contributed a great deal to the misery of insomnia because the insomniac is under the impression that he is getting an even worse deal than is truly the case.

We may well ask why it is that poor sleepers should exaggerate their loss of sleep. In fact it is not necessarily the case that this is a true feature of insomnia. Dr Frankel's selection of patients included only people who had complained of insomnia loudly enough to attract the attention of the medical profession. They were also patients who attributed persistent feelings of irritability, nervousness and excess fatigue to their chronic sleep difficulties. It is to be expected that such patients would pay more attention to, and would remember more, the occasions when they woke during the night because these exasperating events are a reminder of their unhappy day-time state. It is understandable that they will have more vivid and elaborate memories of the waking intervals. But let us not forget that there are many people who normally sleep as badly or worse than the insomniac group in Dr Frankel's study without ever making public complaint and without suffering any nervous debilitation as a result. We do not know anything about their ability to make estimates of the time spent sleeping and waking.

Nevertheless, it is clear that any discussion of the nature of insomnia is clouded by the fact that many insomniacs often think that they are getting less sleep than they really are getting. Moreover they may well have an over-optimistic view of the amount of sleep which other people are getting because good sleepers appear to exaggerate the amount of time spent sleeping. This intensifies the belief, cherished by insomniacs, that they are missing out on a luxury which should be their birthright. It is unlikely that the problems of the insomniac are simply caused by misinformation but they are certainly not helped by it.

Insomnia through misinformation

Some categories of insomnia derive directly from an inadequate appreciation of just how much sleep the body needs. This applies especially to individuals who attempt to get more sleep than they are entitled to. Going to bed early and getting up late is a common pattern among old people, especially if they live alone and have a good deal of time on their hands. If they spend ten hours in bed it is not surprising that they lie awake for two or three hours each night. Their difficulties will be made worse if they take a two-hour nap during the day. A siesta may be relied upon to substantially delay the time of going to sleep at night. Patients confined to bed have a special problem here because the opportunities for day-time sleep are great. The difficulties which such people experience in obtaining a 'good night's sleep' are probably not due to any failure of the sleep control mechanism. They are, more likely, due to its excellent functioning.

Two further examples of insomnia through misinformation arise from the general belief that we need approximately eight hours' sleep per night and that normal sleep leaves you feeling refreshed and eager to begin a new day. In fact, very few people spend eight hours sleeping every night, although they may spend that amount of time in bed. A good average is probably somewhere between seven hours and seven-and-a-half. Unfortunately this statistic is of as little value as the size of an average glove. The amount of sleep which satisfies one is usually very different from that which satisfies another. An inflated view of the 'national average' is probably, in itself, responsible for a great deal of imagined insomnia. The sooner it is deflated, the better.

Similarly, it is also about time that someone exploded the myth that a good sleep causes you to wake refreshed. This is simply not true. Very few people wake up cheerfully. Post-waking nausea is the order of the day for almost everyone. It disappears gradually as the day wears on but it may be especially slow to go if we have nothing to look forward to but the daily chores. Conversely, if we do have something exciting to do, then it may go very quickly indeed. Either way it probably has little to do with the quality of our sleep. Certainly it seems that the nausea which we do feel is accentuated by an excess of sleep - the so-called Rip Van Winkel effect. The best way to avoid it is, first, to have something to look forward to, second, to avoid getting more sleep than you strictly need and, third, to get up at exactly the same time each morning so that the natural body rhythm can synchronise the regular morning upsurge in mood tone to a period immediately after waking.

Insomnia and sleep loss

If, as it seems, there are real difficulties in making subjective judgments concerning the objective quality of our sleep, we should really address ourselves to the question of whether insomniacs really do get less sleep than normals. This question is made all the more pressing by the discovery that insomniacs typically exaggerate their estimates of how much sleep they really do lose.

Unfortunately, there have been few studies to date of the objective sleep of avowed insomniacs. Such studies which do exist indicate that sleep is indeed of poorer quality and of shorter duration but the impairment is not as dramatic as one might expect. For example, in Frankel's study the group of insomniacs averaged only 40 minutes less sleep than normals. This appears to have been largely due to a considerably increased delay in falling asleep. Insomniacs took almost 40 minutes longer than normals to fall asleep. Other measures such as number of awakenings and time spent awake during the night showed only small differences.

Another study which compares good and poor sleepers provides broad confirmation of these results except that poor sleepers on this occasion spent 40 more minutes awake during the night than good sleepers while the delay to falling asleep was only 10 minutes longer. This study was reported by Lawrence Monroe[4] who did not use a clinical population of insomniacs. His poor sleepers were merely college students who reported poor sleep when asked; they certainly did not consider themselves to be suffering from insomnia. Nevertheless, it is interesting to note that his two groups had almost exactly the same amount of sleep as Frankel's two groups.

The picture which emerges from laboratory studies is that insomniacs do have less sleep; they do take longer to fall asleep; they do spend longer awake and they may even wake slightly more often. However, the difference between them and normals is substantially less than we would expect from a simple comparison of their own subjective estimates. These would lead us to expect a difference in sleeping time approaching two hours. In fact the real difference is more likely less than one hour.

These results constitute an intriguing finding since, hitherto, the problem of insomnia has always been viewed in terms of lack of sleep. Certainly it is likely that some insomniacs do suffer regular sleep deprivation, but the bulk enjoy substantially more sleep than we had previously assumed. Once again, it is tempting to dismiss the complaints of insomniacs as exaggerations based upon a germ of truth, but that would be premature. Insomniacs are suffering from something. However, it seems reasonable to ask whether the loss of 40 minutes' sleep is itself an explanation of all the trouble. After all, if a normal healthy volunteer were deprived of 40 minutes of sleep each night, it is most unlikely that he would suffer at all! Perhaps the exaggeration of sleep loss by insomniacs has been a red herring which has misled a medical profession which itself has attached too much importance to the theory that sleep is necessary for restoration purposes. Perhaps this misconception is to blame for the fact that there is currently no satisfactory treatment for the complaint.

Alternative approaches

If the total amount of sleep is not the critical factor in insomnia, what is? One possibility is that poor sleep contains less of some vital ingredient. Monroe's poor sleepers showed 37 minutes less dreaming sleep than good sleepers. Perhaps this is the answer. Unfortunately Frankel's group of chronic insomniacs showed only six minutes less. In any case, we have also seen in chapter 4 that deprivation of dreaming time is no longer believed to lead to any ill-effects. Nor for that matter does the selective deprivation of any particular type of sleep lead to any outbreak of symptoms which we might associate with insomnia. This area has still not been fully explored and we may yet expect some surprises from selective sleep loss studies but at present the consensus is that insomnia does not have its roots in the loss of a particular kind of sleep.

A rather different line of research, which I think is well on target, is being carried out by Mike Herbert at Cambridge University. He took normal volunteers and disturbed their sleep by making the bedroom too hot or by playing sudden loud noises through the night or by forcibly waking them so that they could carry out a short routine task. In the morning he asked them how well they had slept and how often they had woken during the night. His intention was to investigate what caused the volunteer to feel that he had slept badly. He found that reports of poor sleep were unrelated to the amount of different kinds of sleep which the subjects had enjoyed. So far, the only objective guide to what the volunteer will say about his sleep is that a poor quality rating is most likely to be associated with a memory for a large number of awakenings. Mike Herbert[5] makes the point that our perception of the goodness of our sleep is more likely to be based upon an analysis of what we remember about the experience. It follows that feelings of having slept badly must be based upon waking experiences during the night since we remember little of what happened while we were asleep.

These waking experiences are restricted to the period before we fall asleep and those intervals of wakefulness which puncture the continuity of sleep. This brings us full circle back to the sleep instinct which during the night makes being awake an unwanted and unpleasant experience. As a consequence, our memories of a disturbed night are unpleasant memories and we make special efforts to avoid repeating the experience. These efforts, all too often, involve a visit to the doctor to ask for sleeping pills. If our unpleasant night-time experiences persist, we come to long for deep refreshing sleep and release from the regular nightly agony of not being able to slip easily from the world of waking to the world of sleeping.

This is really not a problem of lack of sleep because we do eventually fall asleep and in most cases get a reasonable amount before morning. The problem is really one of spending a long period of time in a state of conflict over which we have little control. Strictly speaking the unpleasantness occurs at a time when we are not sleeping but it would be wrong to conclude that the symptoms of insomnia are caused by sleep deprivation. Some lack of sleep may be involved but in my opinion this is not the major cause of the problem.

This approach does not to do justice to the possibility of any after effects caused by succesive nights of disturbed sleep. While I do believe that the major problem of insomnia is the misery experienced during the night, I agree, none the less, that additional symptoms during the day-time are to be expected. However, these are highly variable and may arise in different ways. Certainly I do not agree that insomnia regularly generates a simple set of persisting after-effects because, as we have seen, the complaints of insomniacs are not highly consistent.

True loss of sleep, when it does occur, might reasonably be expected to lead to sluggishness and a tendency to fall asleep more easily during the next day. For obvious reasons such insomnia is probably only short-lived since sleep will come more easily on the second night. This problem is probably restricted to the occasions where sleep is disturbed by some temporary cause, such as an uncomfortable hotel bed or the arrival of some exciting news. The evidence that we have suggests that this is not the central issue with chronic insomniacs whose sleep, while disturbed, is not chronically less than that of normals, nor do they often complain of excessive sleepiness.

Such individuals may well carry a small sleep deficit forward from night to night but in itself this need not be a great nuisance. Indeed, many insomniacs appear only to complain of their night-time agonies and make little reference to any day-time symptoms. However, it is likely that this residual sleep pressure does interact with other adverse circumstances in some individuals so as to produce a collection of various complaints which are added to the catalogue of night-time miseries. In some cases the unpleasantness of disturbed sleep is superimposed upon a joyless life causing an intensification and focusing of the sufferer's disenchantment with life. Curing the insomnia will not in itself reinvigorate the patient but it could be one less problem to cope with. Other patients may be cases where the disturbed sleep is caused by a pre-existing tendency to worry, to suffer from irrational anxieties, to be tense and irritable and even frankly aggressive. The insomnia will clearly aggravate these conditions and eventually come to be identified wrongly as their major cause.

In the same vein, many people are excessively concerned with the state of their health which they have been educated to believe is threatened by poor sleep. If their health is poor and if they suffer simultaneously from insomnia, it is natural that their disturbed sleep should be held as blameworthy for their ill health. Indeed, there is a germ of truth in this because the persistent frustrations of the night and the small residual sleep deficit will reduce their ability to remain cheerful and positive in the face of adversity. This does not, however, prejudice the fact that insomnia, even when it is persistent, is not generally considered as a cause of ill health.

To summarise, the chronic insomniac is an individual who regularly experiences unpleasant and frustrating conflicts which result from not being able to fall asleep promptly either soon after going to bed or following a spontaneous arousal from sleep. These experiences generate feelings of irritability or depression which may persist into the following day. Disturbed sleep sometimes, but

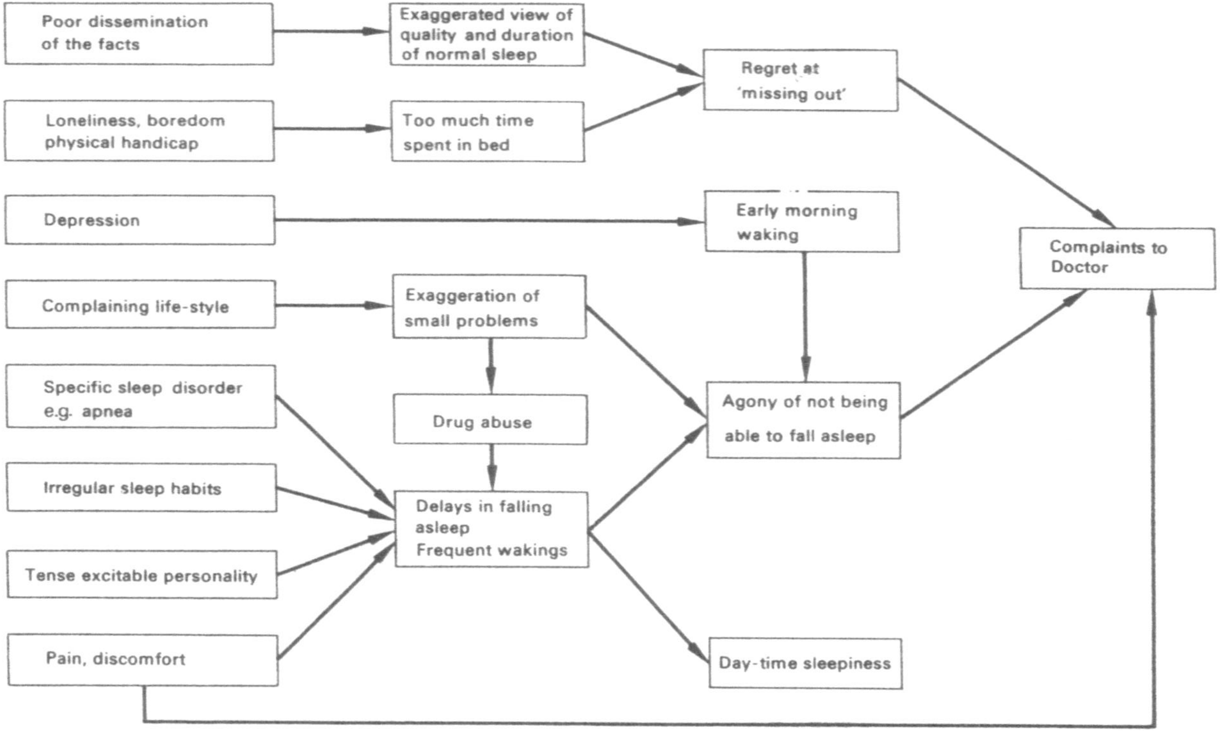

Figure 7.1 The insomnia maze (greatly simplified)

not always, results in a residual sleep pressure which may further depress spontaneity and resilience. These carry-over effects interact with and intensify pre-existing problems, adverse personality deficits or irrational worries concerning the harmfulness of sleep loss. Some pre-existing problem is almost certain to exist as the factor which initially caused the disturbed sleep and the two will become compounded. The loss of substantial amounts of sleep does not itself appear to be a major problem even though, for one reason or another, insomniacs are often under the genuine impression that this is the case.

Treatment procedures

As long as the problem was seen to be one of sleep loss, treatment procedures were relatively straightforward. Administration of barbiturates seemed to be the obvious solution. These are well known to induce long periods of uninterrupted sleep and were prescribed, and still are prescribed in some quarters, in large quantities. Unfortunately experience has shown that this procedure has so many disadvantages that there is now a widespread movement within the medical profession itself to discourage their use.

These problems are various. Perhaps the most serious difficulty arises from the fact that barbiturates when used in high doses have an anaesthetic action and paralyse the lower centres of the brain causing death by interfering with heart and lung functioning. As we know, death from barbiturate overdose, whether intentional or accidental, is only too common. This is, or ought to be, a matter of general public concern. Barbiturate preparations are, of course, addictive drugs which if taken over a long period lead to physiological dependence which is a more severe problem than the symptoms which the treatment was originally intended to deal with. Moreover, the regular use of barbiturates may itself cause, or exacerbate, depressive episodes and suicidal tendencies.

Even the value of barbiturates as a treatment of insomnia has come to be increasingly questioned. The most obvious problem concerns the hangover which many users complain of on the following morning. Feelings of dull lethargy are, after all, the opposite of the desired state of refreshed wakefulness. Recent laboratory studies are also in general agreement that barbiturate induced sleep differs significantly from natural sleep, especially in that dreaming episodes are considerably reduced in length on the first few nights after beginning treatment or after an increase of the regular dosage. The significance of this effect is still not yet generally understood but it should give pause for thought.

The major problem is that the effectiveness of barbiturates is typically short-lived. Patients quickly build up tolerance and their sleep may deteriorate until it is as bad as or worse than before treatment. Some American investigators have even found that they can cure some chronic insomniacs by slowly weaning them from barbiturates. It appears that regular use of these compounds may itself be one of the most potent causes of chronic insomnia in the western world.

Once the hypnotic power of a given barbiturate dose has waned, it can only be regained by increasing the amount taken. The new higher dose will work for a while but quite soon a new increase will be required and the patient will be well on the road to addiction. At this point, the most serious disadvantage of barbiturate use becomes obvious, because a regular user will experience moderate to severe disturbance of sleep for up to a week if he is to sleep without taking his tablets. This means that a patient is not in a position to take or leave his pills. If he does not take them he will experience a few nights of unpleasantness which arise, not from a return of his old insomnia, but from disturbances which are the direct result of biochemical imbalances caused by the withdrawal itself. An alternative to this 'Cold Turkey' approach must involve a medically supervised gradual reduction of the dosage over a period of weeks or months.

In this context we must welcome the arrival of the minor tranquillisers which combine a hypnotic effect with a reduction in tension and anxiety. The use of benzodiazepine drugs in preference to barbiturates has been increasing steadily in recent years because they have proved to be safer and appear to be non-addictive. Since insomnia may often be caused by tension and anxiety, we must welcome any sleeping drug which attacks the causes as well as the symptoms. So far general consensus among sleep researchers is that the benzodiazepines produce sleep which is much more natural than the sedation of barbiturates.

At first sight it seems too good to be true, but, as with all drugs, there are qualifications. So far it is too early to be sure that the drugs are completely safe in the long term and we must remember that most chronic insomniacs will want to take large doses over long periods. Moreover, these drugs will often be mixed with other drugs since insomnia is commonly linked with other complaints. It may be many years before we have a full understanding of the dangers or safety of this mixing. Problems of tolerance associated with long-term use may also prove to be complications.

New horizons

The use of drugs is, of course, not a cure for insomnia; it is merely a treatment which makes it bearable. The complaint may well prove eventually to be beyond a simple cure since its causes often lie deep within the depths of personality which must remain inviolate, but the search for better and better palliatives must continue. In particular the aim must be to find drugs which are effective at ultra-safe low doses and which are carefully aimed at removing sleep disturbance without introducing unnecessary complications into waking experience.

Many insomniacs suffer simply from difficulty in falling asleep at the beginning of the night. After this point, occasional arousals during the sleep period are not especially troublesome. Such sleep onset insomnia may well prove to be best treated by some quick acting drug which merely serves to help them over the first hurdle, causing them to fall asleep but allowing the natural sleep mechanisms to take control thereafter. Such a drug could afford to have only short-lasting effects and might be administered through an inhaler or nasal spray. The advantage of this is that the body is exposed to only very small quantities of the drug and tolerance would be slow to develop – like smoking only half a cigarette a day. This same technique could be used if the patent woke during the night and was unable to fall asleep again. It could not be used to help people get more sleep than they really needed because the body's natural control would fail to keep them asleep and they would wake up again within a few minutes.

This inhalation procedure would probably be of no avail with patients who are suffering from disorders of the sleep control mechanism itself. These would include patients who wake frequently, who have nightmares, who sleep-walk, or who experience respiratory disorders such as asthma or sleep apnea. Hopefully we will be able to develop specific drugs which will tackle these illnesses in a more direct fashion, drugs which result from a thorough understanding of the complaint.

Another completely new approach, which might help these people directly, is suggested by the immobilisation theory itself which admits of the possibility of drugs which will *reduce* the pressure to sleep. Since insomnia is viewed as a conflict between forces which act to make us sleep and forces which act to keep us awake, there are two obvious ways of reducing the intensity of the conflict; either we intensify the sleep inducing forces, thus promoting a straight victory, or we eliminate them thus establishing 'no contest'. The intensification procedure is the traditional technique using sedatives or minor tranquillisers while the elimination of sleep pressures is an approach which has not even been seriously considered by the medical profession nor yet will it be considered so long as the old restoration views hold sway.

As I conceive of the matter, it should be possible to develop a drug which will eliminate temporarily the desire to sleep without creating a sleep debit situation. Such a drug would cure the problems of insomnia, at a stroke. Whether or not it would create additional problems is another matter. We shall only find out by trying. It does seem unlikely that it would prove popular among the regular visitors to the doctor's surgery who complain of sleep disturbance. To them it would appear a strange cure indeed, like treating minor sexual inadequacies by castration. Nevertheless, they may be interested in taking the drug by day, since it would have the effect of reducing the residual sleep pressure left from the previous night. This would make them less tired and possibly make them a little more cheerful if, as many of them believe, their nervous energy is indeed sapped by their drowsy, fatigued condition.

Such a drug would be of more immediate benefit to those individuals, both adults and infants, who suffer apneic attacks – cessation of normal breathing – during sleep. A strong case could be made that some of these individuals would be better off without sleep altogether. Any procedure which eliminated the risk of crib deaths would certainly outweigh the extra care and attention required by a baby at risk which would now be awake for the full twenty-four hours of each day. I am sure that many asthma sufferers would also welcome this treatment. For many of them sleep is full of terror because it carries with it the threat of an agonised and nightmarish awakening from sleep in the grip of an asthmatic attack.

A pill which eliminated sleep pressure would have enormous advantages over the stimulant drugs which merely combat sleep by encouraging the forces which promote wakefulness. In principle, it would have fewer side effects because it will involve fewer bodily systems. It could well be used, in small doses, in any situation where lapses of attention could prove dangerous, such as late-night driving, since it is quite likely that these lapses are caused by the sleep pressure system.

This is not pie-in-the-sky theorising. Recent research has made enormous progress in specifying which parts of the brain are involved in regulating sleep and waking. It has also isolated specific chemicals which are involved in this process. We also know a great deal about how the brain constructs and later destroys these control substances. There is every good reason for hoping that the biochemists and neurophysiologists will soon be able to regulate these processes safely, if they are given suitable encouragement and support.

Drugs will solve some of the problems; the psychologist must tackle others. Some forms of insomnia are the products of misinformation, of outdated theories concerning the need for beauty sleep and misleading pronouncements by the medical profession concerning 'normal' amounts of sleep. A lot of suffering would disappear overnight if people could be convinced that we 'need' only four hours sleep and the rest is a luxury. Even greater benefits would follow from a campaign informing people that it is all a luxury.

At the same time insomniacs must be encouraged to seek an objective measure of just how long they really do sleep. Many will get a pleasant surprise. There is no need to go to a sleep laboratory for this – even if one could be found. Simply place a row of twenty peanuts beside the bed before lying down. Eat one every ten minutes before you fall asleep. Eat one every time you wake up or for every ten minutes you lie awake. In the morning count how many are left and use this number to calculate how much sleep you really did get. If the laboratory findings are to be relied upon, a lot of people are in for a surprise.

The major psychological problem is the unpleasantness of poor quality sleep. If patients could be encouraged to see this simply in terms of a discomfort like backache, many would tolerate it bravely. At present poor sleepers are afraid of the danger to their health of poor sleep and this makes their suffering more acute. They must be reassured. Others are encouraged to exaggerate, to themselves and others, the extent of their suffering because they believe that this is the only way to acquire sleeping pills. There is no obvious solution to this problem except by making the safer tranquillisers more freely available or by publicising their ineffectiveness as a long-term cure and their possible role in making insomnia a permanent condition. As a general rule, anything which causes patients to exaggerate their suffering or to dwell upon their complaint must be minimised. For most people, insomnia is really nothing more than a source of irritation and discomfort, if they are told that it amounts to nothing more they will better be able to keep a proper perspective on the matter and complaints to the doctor, who can't help anyhow, will be minimised.

None of these new horizons will be reached if we persist with the old notion that we need sleep to repair our tired minds and bodies. The sooner this idea is set aside the sooner we can make real progress in minimising the suffering of insomniacs.

8 Review

Whatever people may say, theories are nothing more than ways of looking at things. Certainly the evidence in this book has been collected and presented with the simple aim of influencing the way you, the reader, think about sleep. My aim has been to place sleep in its proper context of complex motivations and organised behaviour. To believe that sleep is simply a blank space - or even a 'unique physiological state' - between going to bed and getting up, is to miss the important fact that sleep is part of an important behaviour control system which influences our thoughts, aspirations and abilities of our everyday working life. Sleeping is behaving just as eating, fighting, socialising and copulating are behaving. In addition I have tried to rid the sleep concept of its centuries old associations with the need for rest and recovery. In my opinion there is no necessary connection between the two. The belief that there is a connection is probably one of the heaviest anchors currently slowing our progress toward more useful theories of the nature and function of sleep.

We can put the controversy into a nutshell by asking whether sleeping has more in common with eating than sexual activity. We know for certain that the purpose of eating is to keep the body in good repair by ingesting necessary food supplies. Sexual activity, on the other hand, is unselfishly concerned with bringing a male's seed to within swimming distance of a female's egg. Both of them resemble sleep in that they call upon powerful instincts which cause the individual to surmount, when necessary, fearsome obstacles so that the drive may be satisfied.

After periods of sustained deprivation of both hunger and sex drives, rebound phenomena occur. The starving man not only eats more, when given the chance, but also eats with much greater vigour than normally. The sex-starved man, likewise, engages in sexual activity in a more sustained and vigorous manner when opportunity finally permits. A sleep-deprived man also sleeps deeper and longer than normal but how shall we explain this? Do we compare him to the hungry man and say that he slept longer because his body needed the sleep? Or do we compare him to the sex-starved man and say that he slept longer because it is in the nature of instincts that they become stronger, the longer they are frustrated? The argument cannot be resolved at this level of armchair theorising but it should be obvious that the traditional comparison of sleep and hunger is not the only possible one.

Sleep and survival

Scientists who study animal behaviour have long been familiar with the idea that sleep is a very useful aspect of behaviour which favours the survival of many species in a way which has nothing to do with the repair of the hurt mind or tired body. They have noticed that most species take great care in the selection of their sleep site and that during sleep they are well protected from most predators and many of the inclemencies of the environment such as extreme heat and cold. It is also obvious that a sleeping animal will waste less energy and water than one which escapes predators by fleeing. From the point of view of survival, sleep is a most advantageous state, an ideal way of spending time not needed for other vital survival activities.

In this connection the sleep instinct offers a number of important services. It causes an animal to sleep for a fixed number of hours each according to how many hours are typically available to that particular species. It also supervises the general business of going to a safe sleep site and adopting a comfortable heat-retaining or heat-dissipating sleep posture. It delays sleep until all of this is satisfactorily arranged. In addition, it takes care to cause the animal to sleep and wake at the most suitable times of day. These features of the sleep instinct are obviously present in man as they are in most members of the animal kingdom. It is difficult not to believe that the most important, if not the only, function of sleep is to schedule behaviour into periods of activity and secluded inactivity.

Carefully adjusted activity-inactivity scheduling is not only vital in normal adults but can be seen clearly at work in babies. They have very little need to be active, since all of their needs are supplied by their mothers. At the same time the mother's job is made much easier if the infant is inactive for most of the time. For many species the survival of the infant may depend very much upon its ability to remain asleep for most of the day. Sleep is also of value in animals which have been injured or infected. When this is the case, it is probably more important to get better soon than to eat. At such times, sleep offers an ideal way of reducing stress to create the best possible conditions for recovery. Sleep need not itself command any special healing powers but it can prevent other strains from slowing the recovery process down. Hibernation offers yet another example of the value of sleep in keeping some species inactive for the duration of a hostile season. No one imagines that the hibernating animal is resting to recover from the exertions of a busy year, although it could conceivably appear so to the animal about to retire for the winter.

Sleep, rest and repair

Perhaps it is these feelings of fatigue which we all experience before retiring in the late evening, which are responsible for the almost universal belief that sleep is a time of rest and recuperation. The very language which we use makes it difficult to think otherwise. We use the work 'tired' to describe our feelings both after heavy physical exertion and in the late evening after a relaxing day in the sun. In the first case, our tiredness is the result of exercise but in the second it is not; we feel tired at midnight every night whether we have extended ourselves physically and mentally or not. Nevertheless, the feelings of tiredness which we have on both occasions are very similar and it is difficult to avoid the subjective assumption that physical and mental exhaustion are responsible for both.

The problem can be seen differently, however, if we accept that feelings of tiredness represent a decision by the brain to discourage further activity. In the case of physical exertion it is important that activity should cease before the point of total exhaustion. Feelings of tiredness compete with the desire to continue the exertion and gradually increase until they finally suppress it altogether. If we are running after a thief, our desire to catch him remains constant while our feelings of fatigue quickly increase in competition until we give up the chase and take a rest (if we have not already caught him). The sleep instinct similarly causes increases in feelings of weariness in order to encourage us to cease whatever we are doing and go to bed. In this case our sense of fatigue does not result directly from the exertions of the day although tiredness from this source may combine to intensify it. The feeling is the same but the source is different. It is understandable that the two should become confused on one's mind but that is hardly a basis for a scientific theory.

It seems quite likely that the subjective feelings of fatigue experienced by scientists themselves before going to bed have had an unfortunate effect on their ability to deal objectively with the available evidence. As a consequence, undue significance has been attached to particular facts which are, in reality, open to various interpretations. For example, after missing a substantial amount of sleep most people will sleep longer on what is misleadingly called a 'recovery night'. In my experience, researchers find this highly suggestive of the existence of a need for sleep in the same sense as a need for food, water and vitamins. Nevertheless, we can observe similar phenomena following all kinds of deprivation without needing to postulate any physiological need. For example, a mother separated from her children will fuss and attend to them more than usual on reunion. Lovers, after a long absence, will engage in courtship activities in a much more intense and prolonged fashion than when they see each other regularly. It is clear that rebound phenomena after deprivation need not indicate any physiological deterioration at all and, yet, so many scientists assume that this must be the case for sleep. The rebound phenomenon is simply being used as a support for their preconceptions, rather than as a piece of evidence in a rational investigation.

It is certainly true that we sleep for approximately the same length of time whether or not we have exerted ourselves on the previous day. Many studies have confirmed this fact. As a result repair theorists have been forced to set aside simple notions of physical fatigue and address themselves instead to poisons, waste products, or strains which accumulate simply by virtue of the fact that we have been awake. According to this idea sleep alternates with wakefulness and sets right the things which have gone wrong and which could not have been put right in the waking state, like a ship which has to be beached for repairs to its hull.

This approach runs up against the difficulties of explaining why different people need different amounts of sleep. Although we sleep on average for roughly seven and a half hours a day, it is quite common for some individuals to take more than nine hours and others less than five. It would therefore not be difficult to find two people in the same neighbourhood, one of whom regularly took twice as much sleep as the other. It could be argued that this situation is analogous to food consumption where some people eat twice as much as others. However, it would be difficult to press this analogy to cover the people introduced in chapter 3 of this book who happily take less than one hour of sleep each day. My belief is that these cases can only be explained if we adopt the view that the amount of sleep taken by individual members of a species is not important. Like sexual activity, it does not matter that individuals do not participate, as long as enough do participate to guarantee the continuation of the species.

The animal studies reviewed in chapter 2 points to a similar conclusion. Mammals show a great deal of variation across species in terms of the amount of sleep they take. Some sleep hardly at all and some sleep nearly all of the time. These differences do not reflect any obvious variations in physiology or amounts of physical activity but they are closely linked to the life style of the species. Animals which can satisfy all of their needs in a few hours each day, fill in the rest of their time with sleep. Other animals, which need to remain awake in order to collect large quantities of food or to be vigilant against predators, seem able to survive with very little, or even no, sleep. Such evidence seems to me to be powerfully in favour of the theory that the sleep instinct merely seems to schedule the activity-inactivity periods of an animal.

It would also seem that the evidence runs counter to recuperation explanations of the function of sleep. However, we cannot be certain of this until someone comes up with a clear and confident statement of what is being repaired. Only then we can get down to the business of refuting repair theories in a satisfactory manner.

Currently, the situation is that almost everyone believes that sleep does permit repair processes which cannot take place during wakefulness but no one knows what these processes are. This is like a murder case where we are convinced that someone has been murdered but we have no idea who the victim is or where the body can be found. The evidence is wholly circumstantial.

In my view, there is no body, no victim and no murder. There is no direct evidence to support the belief that sleep has any direct association with restitutive processes of any kind. Scientists have been misled by the similarity between the feelings of fatigue which follow exercise and those which precede sleep. They have been impressed by the relaxed quality of sleep itself which resembles the normal postures of rest. These have given rise to a set of prejudices which caused a misinterpretation of the rebound phenomenon where people sleep longer when recovering from a loss of sleep. Added to this our language and culture have combined to make it difficult for us to think of sleep as anything other than a period of rest and recovery when in reality it is not so.

The urge to sleep

The interpretation of the results of sleep-deprivation experiments are a special example of how our customary modes of thinking make it difficult for us to treat sleep research data objectively. After many careful experiments we can now be sure that the main effect of sleep loss is to make us very, very sleepy. This may indirectly affect our perceptions, judgment, interest, patience, memory, strength, etc., but we know that lack of sleep probably has no direct effect upon these functions because, when the need arises, our sleep-deprived volunteer can pull himself together and operate normally or even better than normally. The problem is that lack of sleep undermines the motivation of volunteers so that they only want to close their eyes and go to sleep. When engaged on boring tasks their interest quickly wanes, concentration is lost and performance deteriorates. In dangerous or exciting situations, such as occur often in wartime, people can, and do, continue to perform effectively for many days with little or no sleep. Sleep deprivation does not affect our ability to see, hear, calculate, remember, decide and respond; it simply reduces – often powerfully – our motivation to do so. We may consciously decide to overcome our lack of motivation but this is effective only in the short run.

Sleep researchers have moved only slowly to this conclusion and many are still to come. Such is the force of the popular belief that lack of sleep is a denial of some bodily need, that the early results of sleep deprivation were universally hailed as conclusive support for this view. If we starve a man of food, he will surely die, but if we starve a man of sleep, he does not die. No matter how long we continue our vigil, the worst that will happen to him is that he will eventually fall asleep. He will suffer no long-term consequences. In conclusion we can say that the results of these experiments can be understood in terms of the working of a powerful, involuntary sleep instinct, but that they do not necessarily indicate that we need sleep for the purposes of recuperation.

The powerful urge to sleep which can be easily observed in sleep-deprived persons gives us a special insight into the less obvious, but nevertheless decisive, changes in motivation which occur normally just before the appropriate time for going to bed. The sleep motive is in many respects an avoidance drive. When tired we avoid noise, lights, excitement and extremes of all kinds. We retire to a sleep location which is dark, secure and as comfortable as we can make it. This urge competes with and finally dominates other urges. Discomfort, pain, hunger, curiosity, anxiety and loneliness will all delay sleep but they will not conquer it altogether. The gradually increasing urge to sleep will finally still all of these drives until they are freed again when the time for sleeping has passed. In an emergency, however, the sleep urge can usually be delayed for as long as the danger lasts and few animals will be caught napping when cornered by a predator.

The sleep state

It is possible to understand the nature of the sleep state in terms of the same changes of motivation which are responsible for the urge to go to sleep in the first place. If drowsiness is merely the consequence of a lack of interest in anything but going to sleep, then sleep itself may be a lack of interest in anything but *staying* asleep. It is certainly true that sleepers are most uncooperative when attempts are made to wake them. Usually, however, this is attributed to a failure to perceive the arousing stimulus or a failure to understand its true significance. Traditional theories conceive of sleep as a state in which normal working faculties are inoperative. According to the sleep instinct approach, sleep and waking are exactly the same except for one crucial difference: during sleep we show an extreme reluctance to do anything except stay where we are.

Separate state notions of sleep are certainly encouraged by our own introspections. If I try to think back to what happened last night while I was asleep, I can remember nothing. I cannot remember falling asleep, even though I have a clear impression of my lying awake before falling asleep and of my lying awake in the morning irritably contemplating getting up. Subjectively, the difference between waking and sleeping is as great as that between chalk and cheese.

On the other hand we know from experiment that the mind is not blank during this period. Arousals from active sleep (AS) usually result in vivid dream reports. Arousals from quiet sleep (QS) usually result in reports of thinking activity. When I first began as a sleep researcher, I was always amused when volunteer sleepers claimed that they were 'not asleep' even when woken after an hour-long period of deep and movement-free sleep. When pressed, they would usually claim that they had simply been lying thinking. When told of the infallible witness of our recording apparatus, they would simply shrug their shoulders. Perhaps they were right. Perhaps they were awake and our interpretation of brain-wave recordings is at fault or even it may be that sleep and waking states are not as different as we have always thought.

Sleep seems to be a blank period in our life because we remember so little of what took place in our minds at that time. The failure of memory became clearly evident when it was discovered that everyone experienced, every night, more than one hour of vivid dreaming even though few of us can recollect any of it in the following morning. We still do not know why this memory should fail us but it is generally true that we remember clearly only what we want to remember. What we find trivial or irrelevant often leaves no trace. If we consider sleep to be a period of reduced motivation (to do anything other than continue sleeping) then it may be that we attach very little significance to our night-time thoughts which are therefore not remembered. It is possible, however, that we do remember it, in the sense of having put the experiences into a memory store, but that we do not have the means to recall it. Most memories pop automatically into the mind by association when the right key, or trigger stimulus, is presented. In normal waking life these keys may not be available but it is, in my experience, common to hear people exclaim suddenly that something that they have just seen or heard has reminded them of a dream which they had quite forgotten about.

When experimenting in the laboratory I have also been impressed by the speed with which some people can respond to an arousing stimulus even though our recording machinery confirmed that they were asleep. Pressing a button in response to a loud buzzer in less than three seconds is a very common result and experiments in many laboratories have shown that people are able to discriminate between important and unimportant signals in their sleep. It is difficult to believe that, in these subjects, their minds were 'closed down' for the night. We must therefore consider the possibility that slow responses, or a failure to respond at all, can be explained in terms of a motivational change. Such changes can take various forms. We might, for example, realise that we have to wake up to some noise but be very reluctant to do so. Alternatively we might hear the signal but misconstrue its significance as when, in a dream, we imagine that the signal is part of the dream and therefore calls for no action in reality. A third possibility is that we do not register the signal because we are attending to other more important thoughts. This will occur often because, during sleep, any stimulus requiring action, automatically acquires very low interest value and will have difficulty in capturing our attention.

After centuries of thinking that sleep is a state radically different from waking, it is, perhaps, excessive to hope that people will easily accept the idea that sleep and wakefulness are essentially similar except for motivational differences. Nevertheless, such an approach is consistent with the data and helps us to understand facts which were previously set aside. In particular it gives us some insight into the husband insomniac who claims that he 'did not sleep a wink last night' even though his wife reported hearing snores. The typical response of sleep researchers is to say that he did sleep and that scientific recording apparatus, which never lies, could have proved that he did. If sleep and waking are the same thing, except for motivational differences, they could all three - the insomniac, his wife and the sleep recorder - be right.

Dreaming sleep

The discovery of dreaming sleep (AS) proved a stimulant for sleep research in that more scientists were attracted to the field by this novelty. Unfortunately, it did little to help clarify our thoughts concerning the function of sleep. Instead, the problem became even more complex. The reaction of most investigators was to say that we must need dreaming sleep otherwise it would not be there. By analogy with the popular view that sleep was necessary for repair and recuperation, most assumed that AS was needed for some specific type of repair. Because of the association between AS and dreams, theories of mental healing or reorganisation were especially popular for a time. They were supported by early reports that dream-deprivation might cause mental disorders and they have persisted despite the subsequent failure of other researchers to support this claim. The recent discovery that AS exists in many species of birds and mammals, as well as the discovery that AS is most prominent before and soon after birth, have both contributed to a shift in emphasis from mental to neurological aspects of dreaming sleep.

Despite the availability of many ingenious theories, none has attracted widespread acceptance. The net result is that we now have no satisfactory repair function for either AS or QS to carry out. If you believe in the recuperative power of sleep then no doubt you will be confident that two, or more, functions will one day be found. As matters stand there is no real justification for such optimism.

In chapter 7, I have attempted to argue that the alternation of two states of sleep can be understood as a reflection of the way in which the sleep mechanism was constructed in evolutionary history. It is an argument full of technical features which will depend upon future research for full vindication but it is an example of a type of explanation which does not depend at any point on the traditional view that sleep or any of its component parts are required to re-establish some physiological equilibrium. For such theories, the idea that we need to dream is completely redundant.

Briefly, the theory suggests that AS is a state analogous to and descended from reptilian sleep. Because of the major physiological differences between birds and mammals on the one hand and reptiles on the other, AS was found to be inappropriate in warm-blooded animals. In particular, it has been suggested that the reflexes which operate to maintain normal body temperature during waking are inoperative during AS which, of course, is only a problem for warm-blooded birds and mammals. To cope with this threat, it is likely that AS periods were restricted to brief, well-spaced, episodes. I have suggested that, in the course of evolution, a new kind of sleep (QS) was evolved to fill in the gaps between adjacent AS episodes. QS had the advantage of permitting thermoregulation while the combined AS/QS cycle offered, once again, a way of promoting sustained periods of immobility which, as I have already argued, is often of considerable survival value.

Whether or not the theory can be shown to be generally valid – and I am very optimistic that it can – it must be obvious by now that it is possible to construct theories of AS which are both compatible with the available data and with the immobilisation theory of sleep. I am often reminded of the existence of AS by well-meaning critics as if its very existence were itself a knock-down argument against the immobilisation theory and in favour of repair theories. Nothing could be further from the truth. In fact AS may itself contribute the final nail for the coffin of repair theories by making clear the failure of such theories to establish exactly what is being repaired and when.

Implications

Sleep is a matter close to the hearts of all of us, and it is not my intention to arouse anxiety by suggesting that sleep is unnecessary or by implying that it ought to be given up. Even if we had the knowledge and techniques which would be necessary to eliminate the sleep instinct, I would not recommend their widespread use. Like you, I am jealous of my sleep as I am of all other pleasures of the flesh. The pursuit of pleasure is the right of every man and I would be the last person to deny it.

Knowledge, however, is a pleasure in itself. Seeking a proper understanding of all things which affect our everyday life is a reasonable pursuit of all people, and the burden of ignorance is no less heavy when it concerns something as ordinary and familiar as sleep. We can only guess at the suffering experienced by people who are struggling every night to get the seven to eight hours of sleep, despite the inclination of their brains to dictate less, or the disappointments of millions of children forced to lie awake for hours each night because of their parents' natural anxiety to make sure that their child is well rested. Nor can we readily count the cost arising from the actions of the well-meaning family practitioners who prescribed millions of opiates and barbiturate sleeping draughts simply because they were impressed by the need to keep their patients unconscious for at least eight hours a day.

I hope that the new perspective on sleep which the immobilisation theory offers, will percolate into the medical mind and open up new avenues of treatment for various disorders. When the techniques for reducing the desire for sleep become available, they may prove of inestimable value in treating chronic insomnia, narcolepsy, and other sleep disorders such as sleep apnea. As long as we are gripped by the belief that good health presupposes eight hours' sleep a day, these avenues of treatment will be disregarded. This would be a pity because such patients are, in any case, getting very little pleasure from their sleep and would not be sorry to see sleep erased from their life. They could then enjoy the happy and constructive life style of the healthy nonsomniacs we met in chapter 3. Other disorders such as stomach ulcers and heart problems appear to be exacerbated during AS. If this is the case, then prolonged, selective deprivation of AS may be necessary as part of the treatment. If it is generally believed that 'dream deprivation' is bad for you, then no one will even attempt to discover and perfect the techniques for bringing it about and yet another treatment possibility will have been ignored.

Regular insomnia has always been difficult to treat because we have a very poor understanding of the complaint. Some doctors automatically prescribe sleeping tablets in the belief that substantial amounts of sleep are indeed a pre-requisite for good health while other doctors will prescribe nothing in the belief, probably justified, that the patient is getting enough sleep already. Experience has shown that neither approach is very successful and the insomniac returns again and again for treatment. Our slow progress in this area may be due simply to our obsession with the idea that the patient needs more sleep than he is getting. According to the sleep instinct view, he is really suffering from something else, from the conflicting motivational forces which on the one hand are drawing him towards sleep and on the other are keeping him awake. The agony of insomnia is lying awake and wanting to be asleep. Only in very few cases is the insomniac suffering from an overall lack of sleep.

It is difficult to predict exactly how the new perspective will influence treatment procedures but at the very least it will be valuable in relieving the patient of the fear that a lack of sleep is damaging to his or her health. For many people, especially old folk, the problem should be equated with an 'aches and pains' type of ailment and this may remove many of the emotional fears which accumulate in the mind of the chronic insomniac. In serious cases of insomnia it might even prove necessary to remove the desire to sleep altogether. At least then he will not suffer from the pain of trying to go to sleep when other psychic forces are working against this end. Other possibilities include very powerful but short-action drugs which help the patient over the threshold into sleep whenever he feels the need, allowing natural mechanisms to maintain sleep once the process has begun. In principle, these could be used whenever the patient wakes but in practice would more often act as a reassurance and would not be used too often.

If some forms of insomnia can be classed simply as a form of psychic discomfort, rather than the effects of a repair process failure, we are within sight of understanding the frequently encountered link between neuroticism and insomnia. It is clear, of course, that all forms of tension, anxiety or obsessive concern will delay sleep onset and cause the night to be punctuated with awakenings. However, we must also appreciate that many neurotic symptoms are simply exaggerated complaints of regular discomforts. Some people are more given to focusing on their minor ailments and they experience a greater degree of suffering as a consequence. This is a feature of personality which is not readily altered and any treatment of this kind of insomnia will either not be effective or will cause the complaining to be transferred to another ailment. Many general practitioners are well aware of this and deal with the matter accordingly but laboratory investigators seem to be reluctant to make the point clearly that many so-called insomniacs may be suffering from a neurotic disorder rather than the lack of sleep.

No one has so far devised satisfactory treatment procedures for dealing with insomnia or any of the many sleep disorders. The reasons for our slow progress are probably legion. Not least, is the lack of glamour traditionally associated with this branch of medicine, possibly because sleep disorders are rarely lethal (although crib deaths resulting from sleep apnea promise to be a dramatic exception). More recently, interest in sleep disorders has become widespread, as the result of rapid developments of our understanding of the physiology of sleep. Whether we can make sense of our newly acquired information, may depend on our ability to think flexibly when faced with results which challenge our traditional ways of thinking. The ideas discussed in this book are one such response to these challenging findings. If they act as a stepping stone to even better and more useful theories, then they will have served their purpose.

Notes and references

If you are new to the world of sleep research and want to know more about its technicalities, you can do no better than read either, or both, of the following two books.

Webb, W. B. (1975), *Sleep, the Gentle Tyrant*, Prentice-Hall, Englewood Cliffs.

Dement, W. C. (1972), *Some Must Watch while Some Must Sleep*, Stanford Alumni Association, California.

Chapter 1 The joy of sleep

1 Both Webb (1975) and Dement (1972) (see above) reflect the current dissatisfaction among modern sleep researchers with existing theories of the function of sleep.

Chapter 2 The origins of sleep

1 E. S. Tauber, E. D. Weitzman and E. D. Korey, 'Eye movements during behavioural inactivity in certain Bermuda reef fish', *Communications in Behavioural Biology Part A*, 1969, vol. 3, pp. 131-5.
2 G. Moruzzi, 'Sleep and instinctive behaviour', *Archives of Italian Biology*, 1969, vol. 108, pp. 175-216.
3 For a detailed review of such theories consult I. Feinberg, 'Changing concepts of the function of sleep', *Biological Psychiatry*, 1969, vol. 1, pp. 331-48.
4 F. R. Freeman, *Sleep research: A Critical Review*, 1972, Charles Thomas, Springfield Ill.
5 E. S. Tauber, H. P. Roffwarg and E. D. Weitzman, 'Eye movements and EEG activity during sleep in diurnal lizards', *Nature*, 1966, vol. 212, pp. 1612-13.
6 H. Hediger, 'Wie Tiere Schlafen', *Med. Klin.*, 1959, vol. 54, pp. 938-46.
7 Tauber, *et al.*, op. cit.
8 J. Peyrethon and D. Dusan-Peyrethon, 'Etude polygraphique du cycle vieille-sommeil d'un teleosteen (Tinca tinca)', *Comptes Rendues du Société de Biologie*, 1967, vol. 161, pp. 2533-7.

9 F. Strumwasser, 'The cellular basis of behaviour in Aplysia', *Journal of Psychiatric Research,* 1971, vol. 8, pp. 237-57.
10 F. S. Andersen, 'Sleep in moths', *Opuscula Entomologica,* vol. 33, pp. 15-24.
11 H. Hediger, 'Comparative observations on sleep', *Proceedings of the Royal Society of Medicine,* 1969, vol. 62, pp. 153-6.
12 The figures in this table were given me in a personal communication from Truett Allison, Department of Psychology, Yale University. They are based on his analysis of all available reports. References to many of these studies can be found in R. Meddis, 'On the function of sleep', *Animal Behaviour,* 1975, vol. 23, pp. 676-91.

Chapter 3 Very short sleepers

1 According to Webb (1975, p. 131, see above) it may be possible for most of us to reduce our sleep time by up to two hours by an effort of will alone. Beyond that, the nagging desire to take naps or the difficulty of waking in the morning usually prevents further progress.
2 J. G. McCormick, 'Relationship of sleep respiration and anaesthesia in the porpoise - a preliminary report', *Proceedings of the National Academy of Sciences (USA),* 1969, vol. 62, pp. 697-703.
3 Señora Palomino is described in a series of articles in the British national press: *Sunday People,* 22 April 1973; *Sunday Express,* 26 August 1973 (Roy Rutter); *New Reveille,* 22 March 1974 (Peter Weber) with pictures.
4 H. S. Jones and I. Oswald, 'Two cases of healthy insomnia', *Electroencephalography and Clinical Neurophysiology,* 1968, vol. 24, pp. 378-80.
5 A simple description of sleep laboratory procedures and techniques for classifying sleep stages can be found in Webb (1975, see above) on p. 11 *et seq.*
6 R. Meddis, A. J. D. Pearson and G. Langford, 'An extreme case of healthy insomnia', *Electroencephalography and Clinical Neurophysiology,* 1973, vol. 35, pp. 213-14.
7 This case was communicated to me by Dr Eve C. Johnson of the Clinical Research Centre, Harrow, England.
8 This case was presented at the International Sleep Congress in Edinburgh, July 1975. Some of the details were added by Dr Broughton in a personal communication.
9 C. Fischer-Perroudon, 'Total insomnia for many months and the metabolism of serotonin', Thèse de Médecine, 1973, Université Claude Bernard, Lyon I.
10 C. Guilleminault, J. P. Cathala and P. Castaigne, 'Effects of 5HTP on sleep of a patient with a brain stem lesion', *Electroencephalography and Clinical Neurophysiology,* 1973, vol. 34, pp. 177-84.

Chapter 4 Sleep deprivation

1 Webb (1975, see above) p. 125. Dement (1972, see above) p. 13.
2 I. Oswald, *Sleep*, 1974, Penguin, p. 53.
3 J. Horne, 'The biochemical and psychophysiological effects of sleep deprivation in man', *Physiological Psychology* (in preparation).
4 E. L. Hartmann, *The Function of Sleep*, 1973, Yale University Press, New Haven.
5 Oswald, op. cit.
6 M. Jouvet, 'The sleeping brain', *Science Journal*, 1967, vol. 3, pp. 105-10.
7 W. C. Dement, 'The effect of dream deprivation', *Science*, 1960, vol. 131, pp. 1705-7.
8 W. C. Dement, 'The biological role of REM sleep' in A. Kales (ed.), *Sleep: Physiology and Pathology*, 1969, Lippencott, New York.
9 G. W. Vogel, F. C. Thompson Jr, A. Thurmond, D. Geisler, and B. Barrowclough, 'The effect of REM deprivation on depressive syndromes', *Sleep Research*, 1972, vol. 1, p. 167.
10 Dement, op. cit.
11 F. R. Freeman, *Sleep research: A Critical Review*, 1972, Charles Thomas, Springfield, Ill. p. 76.

Chapter 5 Dreaming sleep

1 For the technical details of all aspects of human REM sleep: Webb (1975) (see above).
2 A. Dallaire, P. L. Toutain, and Y. Ruckebusch, 'Sur la périodicité du sommeil paradoxal: faites et hypothèse', *Physiology and Behaviour*, 1974, vol. 13, pp. 395-400.
3 The references to these studies are to be found in R. Meddis, 'On the function of sleep', *Animal Behaviour*, 1975, vol. 23, pp. 676-91.
4 T. Allison, and H. Van Twyver, 'The evolution of sleep', *Natural History*, 1970, vol. 79, pp. 56-65.
5 H. Van Twyver, 'Sleep patterns in five rodent species', *Physiology and Behaviour*, 1969, vol. 4, pp. 901-5.
6 G. W. Langford, R. Meddis and A. J. D. Pearson, 'Spontaneous arousals from sleep in human subjects', *Psychonomic Science*, 1972, vol. 28, pp. 228-30.
7 J. Fauré, in M. Jouvet (ed), 'Aspects anatomofonctionnels de la physiologie du sommeil', *Centre national de la recherche scientifique, Paris*, 1965, vol. 106, pp. 241-83.
8 P. L. Parmeggiani and C. Rabini, 'Sleep and environmental temperature', *Archives of Italian Biology*, 1970, vol. 108, pp. 369-87.
9 G. W. Langford, R. Meddis and A. J. D. Pearson, 'Awakening latency from sleep for meaningful and non-meaningful stimuli', *Psychophysiology*, 1974, vol. 11, pp. 1-5.

10 H. Van Twyver and W. Garrett, 'Arousal threshold in the rat determined by "meaningful" stimuli', *Behavioural Biology*, 1972, vol. 7, pp. 205-15.
11 A. H. Parmelee and E. Stern, 'Development of states in infants', in C. D. Clemente (ed.), *Sleep and the Maturing Nervous System*, 1972, Academic Press, New York.

Chapter 6 The origin of dreaming sleep

1 Good, unbiased reviews of theories of the function of AS are rare. Both Webb (1975) and Dement (1972) (see above) give a flavour of work in this field, however.
2 P. L. Parmeggiani and C. Rabini, 'Sleep and environmental temperature'. *Archives of Italian Biology*, 1970, vol. 108, pp. 369-87.
3 H. C. Heller, S. F. Glotzbach, J. M. Walker and R. J. Berger, 'Sleep and hibernation II: thermoregulation', paper presented to APSS 2nd International Sleep Congress, 1975.
4 T. Allison, H. Van Twyver and W. R. Goff, 'Electrophysiological studies of the echidna *Tachyglossus aculeatus*', *Archives of Italian Biology*, 1972, vol. 110, pp. 145-84.
5 R. J. Berger, 'Bioenergetic functions of sleep', *Federation Proceedings*, 1975, vol. 34, pp. 97-102.
6 In discussion of the paper by A. H. Parmelee and E. Stern 'Development of states in infants', in C. D. Clemente (ed.), *Sleep and the Maturing Nervous System*, 1972 Academic Press, New York.

Chapter 7 Insomnia

1 Dement (1972), p. 73 *et seq* (see above).
2 C. Guilleminault, W. C. Dement and N. Monod, 'Syndrome "mort subite du nourisson" apnées au cours du sommeil', *La Nouvelle Presse médicale*, 19 May 1973.
3 B. L. Frankel, personal communication.
4 L. J. Monroe, 'Psychological and physiological differences between good and poor sleepers', *Journal of Abnormal Psychology*, 1967, vol. 72, pp. 255-64.
5 M. Herbert, 'Some determinants of subjectively rated sleep quality', *British Journal of Psychology*, in press.

Index